# Exposing the Twenty Medical Myths

# Exposing the Twenty Medical Myths

*Why Everything You Know about Health Care Is Wrong and How to Make It Right*

Arthur Garson Jr., MD, and Ryan Holeywell

ROWMAN & LITTLEFIELD
Lanham • Boulder • New York • London

Published by Rowman & Littlefield
An imprint of The Rowman & Littlefield Publishing Group, Inc.
4501 Forbes Boulevard, Suite 200, Lanham, Maryland 20706
www.rowman.com

6 Tinworth Street, London SE11 5AL

British Library Cataloguing in Publication Information Available

**Library of Congress Cataloging-in-Publication Data**

Names: Garson, Arthur, Jr., author. | Holeywell, Ryan, 1985– author.
Title: Exposing the twenty medical myths : why everything you know about health care is wrong and how to make it right / Arthur Garson Jr. and Ryan Holeywell.
Description: Lanham : Rowman & Littlefield, [2019] | Includes bibliographical references and index.
Identifiers: LCCN 2019008881 (print) | LCCN 2019009652 (ebook) | ISBN 9781538131190 (electronic) | ISBN 9781538131183 (cloth : alk. paper)
Subjects: | MESH: Delivery of Health Care | Health Care Reform | Health Policy | United States
Classification: LCC RA425 (ebook) | LCC RA425 (print) | NLM W 84 AA1 | DDC 362.1—dc23
LC record available at https://lccn.loc.gov/2019008881

## UWE E. REINHARDT, PhD

### 1937–2017

We all think of people we would most like to meet. Some say presidents, others basketball players. When I started in health policy, the person I most wanted to meet was Uwe Reinhardt. I didn't know at the time that I had a chance early on and blew it: he started teaching at Princeton two years before I graduated. Fortunately, we met years later serving on the same committee and became fast friends. He and his wife, Tsung-Mei, were charter professors in a yearly live online course I organized. I told the audience when I introduced him from my hotel room in South Africa that there was only one person whom I would stay up until 2 AM to introduce in the eastern time zone, and that was Uwe.

He predicted everything that the United States was going to face in health care—and the solutions—fifteen years in advance. He was brilliant and hilarious. But the reason Ryan and I are dedicating our book to him is that when he spoke, or when he wrote, he made complexities understandable to a wide swath of the public. We hope to have even a smidgen of that effect on the readers of this book.

Arthur Garson Jr., MD, MPH, May 2019

# Contents

# Preface

For years, Americans have heard that our health care "system" is broken. *Never mind the system—what about me?* you may have asked. *Why is health insurance so expensive, and how do I get cheaper insurance that will cover my family? If I can't afford to buy health insurance, how do I get health care? How do I tell if a doctor or hospital is the best for me? Why are my prescription drugs so expensive, and how can I get cheaper ones that still work?* Health care is the top priority of Americans, above the availability of guns, the economy, and the environment. [1]

In this book, you will see that just about everything you thought you knew about health care is wrong. We expose the myths of medicine on which much of this misunderstanding rests. There are plenty of myths out there, and we picked our top twenty to address here. We want you, the reader, to understand not only the *How do I* questions, which are about "me" (for example, *How do I get cheaper insurance?*), but also the *Why* questions, which are broader (such as *Why are my prescription drugs so expensive?*). We write for the general public and intend to remain nonpartisan. After completing this book, readers should have a basic understanding of issues of medical care and health care. In order to solve our health-care problems, we need fresh ideas, and perhaps better-informed readers can supply them. Certainly better understanding the issues at hand will translate to more informed preferences at the ballot box. Because it's when we have a solid basis of fact that we can, as the title says, make it right—together.

Why write this book now? The country continues to be mired in debate about the Affordable Care Act, or "Obamacare," which was enacted by Congress almost a decade before this book was published. The law accomplished the important goal of decreasing the number of uninsured people in this country by nearly twenty million. But it didn't reduce health-care costs for the country, for employers, or for families. Today, one political faction sees the law as something that can be patched up so that it can work even better for more Americans. The other sees the law as flawed from the onset and won't rest until it's either repealed or, at the very least, stripped of all substance. In the meantime, Medicare for all has emerged as a proposed fix for our nation's health-care woes and is increasingly growing in popularity.

Beyond this specific debate, we write this book because of where the country stands on both the price of medical care and our health outcomes. Each year the United States spends more than $10,000 per person on health care, dramatically more than any other developed country spends, even though Americans don't receive better health care than other countries' residents.[2] The spending statistics wouldn't be so alarming if we were the healthiest country on Earth. But the truth is that we aren't anywhere close: our life expectancy ranks forty-third in the world, and our infant-mortality rate ranks fifty-fifth.[3] Americans just aren't getting their money's worth when it comes to health care. Meanwhile, after years of decline, the percentage of uninsured adults under sixty-five is once again climbing, now totaling 15.5 percent of that population as of 2018.[4] Those numbers matter, since the uninsured receive worse health care than the insured and die much earlier than those with insurance.

We know these problems must be solved—and soon. The price of health care continues to rise, and outcomes must improve. But neither politicians nor policy makers are delivering solutions, and in some cases they contribute to the myths busted in this book. We all have a role in making our health and health care better.

We offer special thanks to Carolyn Engelhard, MPA, without whose encouragement we would never have attempted this book. In 2007, she and Arthur Garson coauthored the book *Health Care Half-Truths*, which first gave us the idea to attack health-care myths.[5] Today's questions largely remain the same, but the answers are mostly different.

The opinions expressed in this book are those of the authors and not the Texas Medical Center.

*Chapter One*

# Myth: US Health Care Is the Best in the World

We say it all the time: America is the greatest country on Earth. And in a lot of ways, that's true. We have the largest GDP of any nation and are responsible for a ton of innovation. But when it comes to *health* care, are we really the best? No. What if we had asked whether American *medical* care is the best; would that distinction matter? You bet it does. Unfortunately, we don't rank particularly high there either.

But before exploring how the United States compares to the rest of the world, we need to understand the difference between these two terms. The best way to think of health care is that the term refers to the overall well-being of individuals and populations. The two major measures of health care are life expectancy (how long you live from birth) and infant mortality (death in the first year of life). What affects life expectancy? Some people may wrongly assume that their life expectancy has a lot to do with the type of treatment they get from doctors. But in reality, according to McGinnis and colleagues,[1] about 40 percent of our life expectancy is determined by things we do (or things done to us)—things like smoking, drinking, doing drugs, being obese, being a victim of violence or accidents. Another 30 percent is due to our genetics. Social circumstances (such as living in wealth or poverty) determine 15 percent of our life expectancy, and environmental exposures (whether or not you live around lots of pollution) account for another 5 percent. That leaves just 10 percent of our life expectancy to be determined by "medical care"—the work that doctors, hospitals, and other providers do.

1

The important takeaway here is that *medical care* only represents a sliver of our *health care*, even though these terms are often used interchangeably.

## HEALTH CARE

Our ability to stay healthy and increase our life expectancy is based on a large number of socioeconomic and environmental factors, such as whether we live in poverty or have insurance. These *social determinants of health*, as they are known, are increasingly recognized by the medical community for the vital role they play. We know that medical care really only affects about 10 percent of our health, so if we want to live longer and be healthier, the way to do it isn't by focusing only on improving medical care. It's by doing things like reducing poverty, improving housing conditions, and adopting healthier eating and exercise habits. All the medical care in the world will not fix those issues. The life expectancy of a black male in Harlem is lower than the life expectancy of a man in Bangladesh.[2]

### Life Expectancy

Life expectancy is often used to gauge a country's overall health. At the beginning of the twentieth century, life expectancy in the United States at birth was forty-seven years. Today it is eighty years. Though this improvement is amazing, we still aren't doing as well as much of the rest of the world. The United States ranks forty-third in life expectancy. How can this be in a nation that prides itself on medical innovation and quality of life? The answer lies in the multiple factors that determine the health a nation's people.

#### Social Determinants of Health

According to the World Health Organization, "social determinants of health are the circumstances in which people are born, grow up, live, work and age . . . These circumstances are in turn shaped by a wider set of forces: economics, social policies, and politics."[3] Social determinants of health refer to factors that all play a role in influencing health—factors like income, socioeconomic status, level of education, occupation, education, rural or urban location, gender, or race and ethnicity. While it is tempting to single out certain factors as having the greatest impact on health, most social determinants of health are related to each other. For example, consider ethnicity and race's effect on US life expectancy: Asian Americans have a current life expectancy of 86.5 years, Hispanics 82.8, Caucasians 78.9, and African Americans 74.6. African Americans are more likely than any other racial or ethnic group to develop cancer and are 30 percent more likely to die from it.[4] While whites lose one hundred years per one hundred thousand people under age seventy-five due to homicides, blacks lose more than eight hundred years.

Education is clearly important, too: Those with more than twelve years of education (more than a high school education) can expect to live to eighty-two, whereas for those with twelve or fewer years of education, life expectancy is seventy-five.[5] Lower income levels are associated with higher levels of violent crime and more deaths due to guns, motor-vehicle accidents, and substance abuse.[6] Higher incomes permit increased access to medical care and allow people to afford better housing and live in safer neighborhoods. Have you ever thought about the fact that many people who live in slums don't have an address? As a result, they may not be counted at the time of a national census. They certainly do not receive notification of benefits that could be related to education or health care, such as schools and Medicaid.

Race and social status are both associated with the health of individuals, although it is often difficult to separate the two. No matter how rich or poor a country is, there is a "social gradient" in health and disease: in Europe and the United States, one's occupation, income, and education have all been shown to predict mortality. Those with higher social positions at the top of the socioeconomic scale have better health than those at the bottom. Perhaps it is because those at the "bottom" have less control over their environment and suffer more stress, which is associated with increased risk of heart disease, absence from work, mental illness, and earlier death.

*Behavioral and Environmental Factors*

Smoking, drinking large amounts of alcohol, and obesity are all related to life expectancy. Among all nations in the Organisation for Economic Co-operation and Development—the OECD—the United States is at the bottom (worst) for child mortality: between the ages of fifteen and nineteen, the US death rate from gun homicide is eighty-two times (8,200 percent) higher than in the rest of the OECD, which represents the world's thirty-five most highly developed nations.[7]

The physical environment can bring harm to individuals as well as communities. Pollution in inner cities caused by automobile exhaust is associated with asthma, lung cancer, and heart disease. At the other end of the spectrum, good environments improve individual and community health, providing more opportunities for physical activity, better transportation options, and urban planning. Living in cities that have green space for walking and opportunities for social interaction as part of community living is related to longer life expectancy, particularly in the elderly. For example, elderly people living near a park live longer than those who do not. While a number of factors could be responsible for this difference, an important one is that those near a park walk more than those who do not.[8]

## Health Insurance

Whether one can get access to medical care most definitely influences life expectancy. Patients can face challenges with access, coverage, or both. *Access* refers to the ability to see a practitioner, such as a physician or a nurse, at the right time and the right place (like by video or e-mail, as not all patients need to be "seen" in person in the office to receive appropriate medical care). *Coverage* refers to whether a person has insurance. An example of access with no coverage is when a patient goes to the emergency department, which is legally required to care for patients, even if they don't have insurance. As for having perfect coverage with no access, consider people in rural areas who are covered by Medicare but have no practitioners. Having access is often related to having insurance coverage. There is a strong relationship between having health insurance and life expectancy. Uninsured adults younger than age sixty-five die at a rate 40 percent higher than those with health insurance.[9]

## Genetics

When we die, how we die, and what we die of are all related to genetics—the DNA code we inherit from our ancestors. We can learn a lot about genetics by studying those who are fortunate enough to have good genes: those who live to be one hundred or more. They represent only one in six thousand people, and it turns out that they fall into nineteen specific subgroups based on genetics. Some of those groups are associated with things like delayed onset of age-related diseases like dementia, hypertension, and cardiovascular disease. (Of course, genetics and the environment are closely related;[10] some smokers never get lung cancer.) Health policy can't do much to improve people's genetics. However, it is now just becoming possible to change one's genes, and these issues will be hotly debated.

## Advances in Public Health

Many people take advances in public health for granted. But in fact these are more important to increasing life expectancy than even medical care. It's the work of public health that led to the recognition of the link between smoking and lung cancer and other lung diseases, to vaccination for diseases such as polio, to motor-vehicle safety (e.g., seatbelts, airbags), to safer and healthier foods, to fluoridation of drinking water.[11] And it's improvements in public health that have helped us understand risk factors like high blood pressure and the importance of exercise in the prevention of coronary heart disease and stroke.

## Medical Care

The last determinant of life expectancy is medical care—or what happens inside the doctor's office or hospital. To a large extent medical care is measured by how well people recover from illness and the likelihood that they stay healthy after treatment. (We'll deal more with medical care later in this chapter.)

Remember—medical care only changes life expectancy by about 10 percent. Therefore improvements in quality of medical care alone have a limited impact in reducing early deaths over the whole population. Why do we keep emphasizing this point? It's not to say that improving medical care is unimportant. But if we want to get serious about improving health—of individuals, of communities, and of entire nations—we have to do more than just focus on improving medical care. We need to change unhealthy behaviors, improve the environment, address poverty, and ensure that people can actually use the medical care that exists. Early in his practice, Dr. Garson met and treated a little girl named Ginny who suffered from a heart condition that was manageable but only with the right medications. Ginny grew into a lovely young lady. But, tragically, she died before her twentieth birthday because her Medicaid coverage had expired and she could not pay for the medications that kept her alive. Ginny didn't die because medical treatment wasn't available for her heart condition. She died because she was uninsured and couldn't afford her drugs.

Finally, it is worth our mentioning that the deaths due to terrorism are now counted separately among all causes of death.[12] Clearly terrorism has nothing do with medical care but a lot to do with larger social factors, illustrating why life expectancy is more an index of health care than medical care.

## Infant Mortality

The infant-mortality rate is the percentage of infants who die in their first year of life. The United States' infant-mortality rate ranks fifty-fifth in the world, tied with Serbia. Infants die in the United States at almost three times the rate as in Japan and at nearly double the rate of South Korea. [13]

Low birth weight and premature birth, as well as birth defects, are responsible for a large part of newborn deaths in the United States. The data, it should be noted, aren't perfect: some countries don't count extremely premature infants and those with very low birth weight. Nonetheless, when a comparison is done of only infant mortality in groups with similar birth weight, there is still higher mortality in the United States. [14]

The United States has the highest rate of teen pregnancies in the developed world, and we know that younger mothers have more premature babies with low birth weight. [15] But we also know that cigarette smoking and alcohol are factors contributing to low birth weight. In addition, higher infant mortality occurs in inner cities and among the uninsured. Racial and ethnic differences in infant mortality are found throughout the developed world and add to other factors, such as smoking and age of the mother. In one US study, African American babies had 1.6 times the infant mortality of Caucasian babies, and those with low socioeconomic status had an infant-mortality rate 1.6 times higher. The mortality for black babies with low socioeconomic status was the highest of all. [16]

Much of this discussion revolves around death in the first month of life—so-called "neonatal" mortality. But infant mortality goes to one year of age. Here the United States also fares worse than Europe. The most common causes of infant mortality after the first month are sudden infant death syndrome—now called *sudden unexpected infant death*—and accidents. Infants may also die from conditions that present at birth but don't cause death until after one month—such as breathing problems and birth defects. [17]

### Prenatal Care

Where does prenatal care figure in to infant-mortality rates? While impactful and important, prenatal care—medical care—affects infant mortality much less than you might think, because social determinants of health, race, and behaviors like smoking, substance abuse, and poor nutrition are also related to birth outcomes.[18] As you can imagine, the data are just as murky as life expectancy: those with low socioeconomic status also have less prenatal care. The conclusion is that some prenatal care is better than none, but at best 10–15 percent of infant mortality is changed by prenatal care.[19] Prenatal care is more likely to improve infant mortality in those with higher risk factors, such as drug abusers.

## WHAT TO DO?

It is important that we continue to pursue long-term answers in our attempts to decrease the infant-mortality rate in the United States. But, as with life expectancy, our best near-term improvements are likely to be achieved targeting social and behavioral factors. Lowering teenage-pregnancy rates, along with reducing maternal smoking, drug and alcohol abuse, and poor nutrition, will go a long way toward improving the health of mothers and newborns. Not only will lowering teen-pregnancy rates improve infant mortality, but it will also improve life expectancy; remember, the death of an infant counts in life expectancy. Most of Europe "has policies for infants between one month and one year, which bring nurses or other health professionals to visit parents and infants at home. These visits combine well-baby checkups with caregiver advice and support and, importantly, reduce infant mortality."[20]

## MEDICAL CARE AND HEALTH CARE

*Medical care* is best defined as what practitioners and patients *do*. Physicians and other medical professionals certainly take care of the sick by providing medicine, performing procedures, and working with them to implement lifestyle changes. Increasingly, they're also being held accountable for keeping people well. Not only are they being tasked to provide counseling and helping with disease prevention, but the results of those efforts are also being measured, such as the percentage of their patients who stop smoking and avoid obesity.

Medical care can be assessed by a number of outcomes such as survival rates for patients with diseases like cancer in adults and childhood asthma in children. An overall index of medical care is the *amenable mortality*—or the "measure of deaths before age seventy-five that could potentially have been prevented by timely access to appropriate medical care."[21] Some preventable deaths include those from tuberculosis, maternal mortality, colon cancer, breast cancer, appendicitis, ischemic heart disease, diabetes, epilepsy, injuries, and medical errors.[22] You may be thinking that it's in medical care that the United States shines. That's not exactly true. In fact, we rank last in amenable mortality among sixteen high-income countries.[23] The United States performs well on cancer care (and has the best breast cancer mortality in the world) but has high rates of mortality from heart disease and amputations as a result of diabetes.[24] Unfortunately, the number of areas in which the United States performs well is outweighed by the areas in which we compare poorly to other wealthy nations.

Many readers will be shocked by these statistics. After all, the United States has some of the greatest medical centers in the world; in fact, both authors of this book work in one, the Texas Medical Center in Houston, with twenty-six hospitals and four medical schools on its campus. But many of these preventable deaths are in people who live in the slums near the medical center and have no health insurance or who live 150 miles from the nearest practitioner. Despite our nation's history of effective and innovative medical treatments, our system of medical care can perform better.

In summary, the United States is a complex blend of different cultures; it's what makes us great and strong. While it may be tempting to "adjust" statistics like infant mortality or life expectancy to take into account people who live in high-crime areas or who have extremely low incomes, that would be a mistake. We should not excuse or explain away our health-care problems but, rather, begin to attack them through improving our social determinants of health. We can most definitely improve our medical care as well, but improving *health* care may prove to be the more effective way to improve and extend lives.

An important postscript: We have pointed out the difference between medical care and health care. This is an important distinction when considering both together. But most people use *health care* when they are referring to either one—such as in the next chapter, where we discuss "national health expenditures," which should really be "national *medical* expenditures." This is not a battle worth fighting, and so you will see us mainly use *health* throughout the book in a nod to current usage. But you now know better.

## CHAPTER SUMMARY

- The distinction between health care and medical care is extremely important.
- In the two metrics of "health care," the United States scores poorly, both in our life expectancy (forty-third in the world) and in infant mortality (fifty-fifth in the world).
- Only 10 percent of our life expectancy is based on the quality of our "medical care"—what patients, doctors, and hospitals do. But we don't rank very highly on that either.

  - Medical-care measures include outcomes of diseases and prevention of disease. By one important measure, the United States ranks sixteen out of sixteen (worst) among developed nations on the number of premature deaths that could have been prevented by timely access to medical care.

- These factors are part of the reason why the life expectancy for a black male in Harlem is lower than the life expectancy for a man in Bangladesh.
- How can it be that we have the greatest medical centers and innovation and the worst overall results among industrialized nations?

  - Nearly thirty million people in the United States are uninsured, and we have a death rate due to gun homicides that's eighty-two times that of other developed nations. That's health care.

- Because most people say *health care* when they mean *medical care*, throughout this book we sometimes use the popular, if less accurate, terminology in a nod to common parlance—as in chapter 2, for example, when we discuss "national *health* care," which readers now understand would be most properly termed "national *medical* care."

*Chapter Two*

# Myth: In Many Ways, US Health Care Is Cheaper than Other Countries'

We have just seen in chapter 1 that there are important differences between *health* care and *medical* care. Health care is broad and includes "social determinants of health" such as poverty.[1]

In the United States we spend a lot on medical care. If you've ever gotten an MRI in the United States, you might (or might not) know that it costs more—vastly more—than the same exam costs in other parts of the world. Your American MRI can cost more than $3,000. In Australia, the price tag is just $215. And, by the way, that American MRI isn't five times "better" than the Australian one. It happens with surgeries too: Hip replacements in the United States cost $29,000 on average—nearly 80 percent more than they cost in the United Kingdom. You could have four appendectomies in Australia for less money than it costs to get one done in the United States. But there's another reason for the high costs: the sheer volume of stuff we have done. Americans undergo MRI exams at almost triple the rate Australians. We get knee replacements 45 percent more often than the French.[2]

Remember, in this chapter we are speaking about *health care*. Our purpose in this chapter is to see whether our health care in the United States, which includes our medical care, is actually cheaper than other countries' health care.

## SOCIAL SPENDING

In order to understand what we and other countries spend, we begin by examining *social spending*, which is both public and private payment to households for support during tough times. This support is not only for medical care but also for payments to individuals for unemployment, housing, and other needs. We know, for example, that unemployment payments can affect more than the recipient's health, but overall social spending gives us a way to compare US spending with other countries' spending. We do this by comparing the percent of the gross domestic product. GDP percentage, by definition, must total at 100, and so the percent of GDP spent in different programs tells what is most important to that country. For social spending *without* medical care, the United States spends 37 percent of GDP, whereas countries in the European Union spend considerably more, at 43 percent.[3] But what happens when we add medical care?

### Medical-Care Spending

The US and EU governments both spend about 8.1 percent of GDP on medical care. But the United States adds another 9.0 percent to that total—what is spent with private insurers—while the European Union only adds another 2.3 percent for private insurers. In total, that means US medical-care spending is about 17.1 percent of GDP, compared to 10.4 percent for the European Union.[4]

While percent of GDP is used frequently to compare countries' spending priorities, a more meaningful measure is the amount of money each country spends on medical care, what is called *national health expenditures*—or NHE. As you know from chapter 1, a more accurate term would be *national medical expenditure*, but here we cave to historical terminology. The most recent NHE for the United States totaled almost $3.3 trillion.[5] We can further break down where, exactly, that spending went. For each health-care dollar spent in the United States, thirty-two cents purchased hospital care, twenty cents paid for physicians and other clinical services, ten cents purchased prescription drugs, and the remaining thirty-eight cents went to various other services such as program administration, home health care, and dental care.[6] The most recent NHE spending *per person* in the United States was $10,348—about 31 percent higher than in Switzerland, the next-highest per capita spender, and exactly twice the amount of the average for other industrialized countries.[7]

There are six reasons why US medical-care spending dwarfs that of its peers, no matter what measure you use.[8]

## US Wealth Elevates US Health-Care Costs

According to recent analysis,

> The health care systems of nations go through three stages as they develop. Low-income countries spend the least on health, and the sources of that little bit of funding are international donors who fund care, as well as residents who spend out-of-pocket. In middle-income countries, residents still pay out-of-pocket, but the government has more capacity to play a role, and thus it pays for some health care. In high-income countries, the money for health care mostly comes from the government and private insurance. Moreover, it follows that those countries with the highest GDPs and the greatest level of spending have people who request more health care.[9]

Clearly the ability to pay for medical care will affect the amount one consumes, and so it is no surprise that the United States has a larger appetite for medical care by nature of its wealth.

The actual level of GDP as a measure of a country's wealth may provide a partial explanation for why the United States and the European Union have higher health spending than, say, Costa Rica. But GDP does not explain why the United States has higher health spending than the European Union. The following five explanations will clarify this issue.

## Our Lack of Bargaining Power Means We Pay More for Less

Virtually all other countries have a single public health-care system that, with great bargaining power, sets prices for all medical care within its borders, including the amounts that will be paid for physicians, hospitals, and drugs. The United States' mostly private, fragmented system allows medical technology and new medicines to come to physicians and patients more quickly, and they are used more often. But that culture of innovation comes at a price.

The Medicare Modernization Act of 2003 prohibits Medicare—the federally funded insurance program for those over age sixty-five—from bargaining with drug manufacturers. The law prevents this massive federal program from using its purchasing power to negotiate for lower prices.[10] Think about it this way: When you go to your local car dealership to buy a pickup truck, you might be able to get yourself a deal, but you probably aren't going to have that much power to dent the price, no matter how skilled a negotiator you are. But say you're a large construction company, and you want to buy hundreds of trucks from that dealer. You might have the power to make or break the dealership's bottom line for the quarter or even the year. Suddenly you're going to have a lot more bargaining power in the negotiation. The dealer would probably cut your construction company a deal, since making less profit on each individual truck is worth it if it means selling more of them in the end. In the United States, we've passed a law that prevents us from using that power.

## *The US Government Isn't Permitted to Consider Cost in What It Covers, Driving Prices Up*

Other industrialized countries weigh the costs of new technologies along with the benefits, which slows the introduction of new medicines and treatments. For example, the United Kingdom has a nongovernmental body, the National Institute for Health and Care Excellence—or NICE—that determines whether and how much the National Health Service will pay for drugs.[11] NICE measures *cost effectiveness*—a mathematical measure of the cost divided by the benefit in years of life. NICE is less likely to pay for certain drugs that are very expensive and thought to be "of little benefit." Naturally, US pharmaceutical manufacturers oppose such a system for use in the United States, claiming that new medical advances would be delayed. Our legislators literally "bought in" to those claims. In 2010, the Affordable Care Act began preventing the federal government from using the cost of care, as well as information about the cost effectiveness of care, in Medicare-coverage decisions. In other words, the government can't say a treatment or drug is too expensive to pay for, given the benefit it provides.[12] At a recent convening of health-policy experts we organized at the Texas Medical Center, we compared this regulation outlawing weighing cost and effectiveness to a "pair of handcuffs"; this situation has to change.

## *Administrative Complexity Creates Waste*

Administrative costs account for 25 percent of total US hospital spending, according to a study that compares these costs across other countries—like England, where administrative costs are 16 percent, and Canada, where administrative costs are just 12 percent. Reducing US spending for hospital administration to Canadian levels would save more than $150 billion every year.[13] If we have numerous insurance companies—each having their own performance measures and billing systems—an administrative nightmare is guaranteed. We consider this problem extensively in chapters 3 and 16.

## The US Concentration on Profits Ends Up Costing Us Money

No other country has the widespread, for-profit organizational arrangements in health care that the United States has. Many health-related organizations in the United States—including insurance companies, most pharmaceutical companies and device makers, and many hospitals—are private and for-profit, and sometimes their stocks are traded publicly. Even the "not-for-profits" in the United States, including hospitals, act like for-profit companies and give bonuses to their executives based on financial performance. This is not necessarily wrong, but it does help to explain why medical costs in the United States are so high.

A large portion of the US health-care system is specifically designed to maximize the cost that can be paid, while most other health-care systems are specifically designed to minimize costs. Some of this entrepreneurialism is cultural: That's just the way we are. This cultural bent—which we'll discuss in greater depth in chapter 17—promotes and permits larger payments throughout the health-care system. In a landmark 2003 article, Anderson and colleagues show that "It's the prices, stupid." Consider, for example, that physicians in the United States are paid around three times more than physicians in other developed countries, and hospital payments in the United States are also about three times higher. Spending on pharmaceuticals in the United States, furthermore, is two to three times that in Europe and Canada because the prices in the United States are higher—not because we use more drugs, which we do not.[14]

## The United States Wastes $1 Trillion per Year on Medical Care

Our overall cost of US medical care is higher than elsewhere in the world, but it's not the number of doctors, nurses, or hospitalizations that drive up cost for us. In fact, in the United States we have fewer physicians, hospital beds, annual doctor visits, and annual hospital discharges per capita than industrialized Europe.[15] The problem in the United States isn't that we go to the doctor or hospital too much. It's largely that we waste $1 trillion in medical spending per year. This is not a guesstimate. Donald M. Berwick, Obama-era administrator of Medicare and Medicaid, calculated waste, which he defines as processes, products, and services that do not help customers. He found, for example, that $200 billion are wasted every year in overtreatment—a topic we'll discuss in greater depth in chapter 3. [16]

## THE BOTTOM LINE: HEALTH-CARE SPENDING

When all social spending—including medical care—is considered by country, the United States is second from the top in the world, at 28.8 percent of GDP. Only France is higher, at 31.3 percent. [17] So, it is a myth that the United States spends the most on *health care*. This is barely the case. But the way we spend the money is vastly different. We surely spend the most on *medical care*, whereas France spends much less.

Our recurring theme is this: Despite leading the world in medical-care spending, the United States has worse outcomes to show for it. One metric is years of life lost per one hundred thousand people. [18] The metric is based on the idea that with the best care there would be no years of life lost. In all countries but one, there is a strong relationship between years of life lost in a country and average medical-care spending per person. Generally, the lower the spending, the greater the years of life lost. Among industrialized nations, the greatest numbers of years of life lost are in Mexico—nine thousand years lost per one hundred thousand people. That's no coincidence, since Mexico has the lowest per-person spending on medical care in the developed world, at about $1,000. The "best" is Norway, with three thousand years lost and spending of $5,000 per person.

However, the United States is the only country that is off the charts in terms of spending. It outspends everyone—$10,000 per person—with an enormous 4,500 years lost per one hundred thousand people. It doesn't take an economist to understand that when you pay three times the amount that somebody else pays for worse results, you're getting ripped off.

## CHAPTER SUMMARY

- Total *health-care spending* includes social spending and medical-care spending. The United States is at the top of the heap in total health spending, second only to France.
- *Medical-care spending* per person in the United States was $10,348 in 2016, about 31 percent higher than spending in the next highest country—Switzerland—and exactly twice the amount of the average for other industrialized countries.

- There are six reasons why the United States spending is so high, and none of them are because we provide the best medical care and get the best medical outcomes.

  - The United States is wealthy, and people in wealthier countries spend more on medical care.
  - The United States has no ability to use its bargaining power to negotiate on behalf of most citizens the way other countries do.
  - The US government is not permitted to consider cost in what it pays for.
  - The US system is weighted down in administrative complexity.
  - The United States has a unique emphasis on profits: "It's the prices, stupid."
  - The United States wastes $1 trillion per year on medical care.

- We spend a lot on medical care without enough to show for it.
- It doesn't take an economist to understand that paying three times as much for worse results is a bad deal.

*Chapter Three*

# Myth: The United States Wastes One in Every Ten Medical-Care Dollars

Huntington, West Virginia, and San Francisco aren't very similar places. If you were asked to list differences, you might start with the view. But the two cities have another key difference: Huntington's cardiologists are some of the busiest in the nation. More than ninety-one out of every one thousand Medicare patients in the region have undergone cardiac catheterization, a procedure in which a tube is inserted into part of the heart to diagnose or treat cardiac problems. In San Francisco, by contrast, the catheterization rate is thirteen out of every one thousand. So why are residents of Huntington getting the procedure at seven times the rate of San Franciscans? It's not because they're sicker. In fact, it's likely that many in Huntington didn't need the procedure in the first place. What's happening is the West Virginians are being *overtreated* and getting care they likely don't need.[1] This is an example of *physician-induced demand*, where physicians recommend treatment that improves their out incomes—and patients dutifully do what the doctor suggests.

Other examples like this abound. Garson recalls the time he was in the waiting room of a doctor's office. He overheard the doctor speaking with a salesman who was selling him an expensive piece of imaging equipment. The two forgot to shut the door during their meeting. "You'll have to do at least seven of these per day in order to make money," the salesman said. "No problem," the doctor replied, leaving the entire waiting room aghast.

These stories bare only the tip of the iceberg, as we will see. You've almost certainly experienced more subtle forms of "overtreatment" in the

19

form of *administrative waste*. You know what happens when you make an appointment with a doctor for the first time: First, you give all your information to a clerk on the phone, who takes down your name, your insurance information, your symptoms, and other information. Then, when you get to the doctor's office, you give it to the front desk again. Then, when you're brought to the examination room, you repeat it all to the nurse yet again. It's not just annoying; it's also a waste of your money. You're paying for that same task to be repeated over and over again.

## HOW DO WE WASTE MONEY?

How much waste is there? According to Donald Berwick, administrator of Medicare and Medicaid during the Obama administration, in order to reduce waste, the US medical-care system would have to modify itself "to keep processes, products, and services that actually help customers and systematically remove the elements of work that do not . . . The challenge in removing waste from US health care will be to construct sound and respectful pathways of transition from business models addicted to doing more and more to ones that do only what really helps."[2]

Berwick found that waste accounts for about a third of the dollars spent on medical care in the United States today; that represents about $1 trillion annually. That's a million-million dollars. The vast wasteful expense isn't just frustrating because it's inefficient but also because there are already limited dollars to spend on health care, and in this country we fight viciously over how to spend them. To put these numbers into perspective, the cost to cover the uninsured is between $150 and $200 billion per year; if we could save just 15–20 percent of the waste, we could cover the uninsured.[3] Table 3.1 shows Berwick's data and gives us a better idea of exactly where our wasted dollars go in a typical year. This paper was published in 2012 and so in 2019 dollars, the total is more than $1 trillion wasted. And now we can explore each of these categories in greater depth.

### Administrative Waste

The United States has a vast bureaucracy to handle billing. Duke University Hospital, where Garson once worked, had 1,300 billing clerks but just nine hundred hospital beds. Overseas, a hospital that size would typically have fewer than ten people working in billing.[4] In the United States, there are a

**Table 3.1.**

| Type of waste | Cost (in $US) |
| --- | --- |
| Administrative waste: inefficient billing procedures | $248 billion |
| Overtreatment: ordering unnecessary tests and procedures | $192 billion |
| Fraud and abuse: overbilling | $177 billion |
| Pricing failures: higher than the rest of the world | $131 billion |
| Failures of care delivery: safety | $128 billion |
| Failures of care coordination: readmissions | $35 billion |
| Total waste | $911 billion |

large number of insurers, each of which requires different information from physicians and hospitals, and each of which has different processes to pay for different medical procedures for different types of patients.

As part of the process, the patient is mailed an *explanation of benefits* from their insurance company (which usually says "This is not a bill," to the confusion of consumers). The form generally is difficult to understand, and patients can't figure out what their insurance will cover, especially because the same form often shows up repeatedly with different numbers. Undoubtedly, an army of insurance clerks exists to process those forms and answer innumerable questions patients have about them.

Part of our inefficiency is having electronic health records—or EHRs—that are not yet as helpful as they could be. For example, practitioners and their staff end up spending a great deal of time on data entry, putting patient information into charts, or otherwise end up on the phone with the insurance companies, trying to get permission to do tests and procedures. And sometimes with this "time-saving" software, practitioners can't figure out how to access existing information, meaning that they might end up ordering a repeat test because they can't find the patient results from the first one, or the data from the location where the test was done is not available in the EHR. In the worst of examples, even within a single hospital (the same building) the tests from one lab may not be available to another.

Administrative costs account for 25 percent of hospital spending in the United States—more than double the spending in Canada, which accounts for 12 percent of their annual spending.[5] Private US insurance companies spend 12–18 percent annually on administration, whereas Medicare spends only 1.4 percent.[6] It is tempting to say that "EHRs can fix all that," and in time that is likely to be true; eventually the software will improve to streamline the vast stores of patient information. But one reason the United States may not be not moving faster to cut administrative waste is that increased efficiency will actually reduce or eliminate jobs. This is not a good reason to keep inefficiency, and we should begin job training people who will lose their jobs in the next several years.

## Overtreatment

Berwick defines *overtreatment* as "the waste that comes from subjecting patients to care that, according to sound science and the patients' own preferences, cannot possibly help them—care rooted in outmoded habits, and ignoring science."[7] More bluntly, physicians perform procedures and tests that are unnecessary. Part of this story involves the overprescription of opioids that have come to dominate daily headlines. Harvard studied this issue and concluded that physicians who prescribe large amounts of opioids are signed up by drug manufacturers for lucrative speaking engagements; thus, the study finds, these doctors are actually being paid to prescribe.[8]

Patients have specific requests for medications and procedures they've seen on the Internet or television or heard about from a friend—so-called *patient-induced demand*. "For a variety of reasons, it's really hard for doctors to say no to patient requests."[9] Patient-induced demand also occurs when a person with a simple condition like a cold visits their physician's office or even goes to the emergency room for treatment. Many times, especially toward the end of a patient's life, better treatment actually means doing less. Patients don't necessarily want complicated, expensive interventions that are unlikely to do any good, but physicians often have a difficult time choosing to do less—a problem we'll discuss further in the next chapter.

Another potential area of waste due to overtreatment is the fear of malpractice. Certainly practitioners see patients more frequently, order more tests, or even perform more procedures because they're worried about being sued; this is called *defensive medicine*. Though there is less of this day-to-day worrying by physicians than you might think or read about in the press, it's still a problem. We'll discuss malpractice in greater detail in chapter 10.

Physician groups know that overtreatment occurs, and in an attempt to curb it, the American Board of Internal Medicine created the Choosing Wisely program, in which more than seventy professional societies, such as the radiologists, create list of procedures or tests that should never be performed on a patient. But a recent review found that of the physician groups in

Choosing Wisely, "at least some omitted services that the practitioners frequently performed."[10] In other words, the program urged practitioners to stop performing procedures they weren't much performing anyway, decreasing the program's effectiveness. Medicare is also working to curb overtreatment by developing ways to pay physicians without rewarding increased volumes of services, such as by salary as opposed to a fee-for-service model.[11]

The late John Eisenberg, who led the federal agency that monitors healthcare safety and quality, offered an important insight into the issue of waste. He said, "to suggest that medical decision making can be divorced from consideration of cost denigrates the complexity of patient care . . . Almost all clinicians would agree that, at some point, the extra money spent on tiny improvements in clinical outcomes is not worthwhile and represents inappropriate practice."[12]

David Eddy, physician and mathematician, helps us further: "In a field filled with uncertainty and doubt," he says, "the difference between 'When in doubt, do it' and 'When in doubt, stop' could easily swing $100 billion a year."[13]

Fortunately, we have a way to analyze tests and treatments that uses relatively simple math. We divide the cost of a treatment by the *added years of life* that a specific treatment will give someone. For example, a coronary bypass surgery that costs $50,000 increases the average length of life by ten years. What we call the *cost-effectiveness ratio* is $5,000 per saved life year. A lower cost-effectiveness ratio represents a better value. For example, that bypass is a pretty good deal, considering that airbags in cars cost about $100,000 per saved life year.

But not every year of life saved is of the same quality. Chemotherapy might add years of life, for example, but some of those years will be full of side effects. In such a case, we would use *quality-adjusted life years*—or QALYs—to take into account those less-than-perfect years. The point is that, by comparing cost of care to how well it works, we have a good idea of how cost effective that care is, especially when compared to other treatments.

Common procedures performed every day, such as coronary bypass surgery or hysterectomies, generally have cost-effectiveness ratios of less than $50,000 per life year. Remember, lower numbers are better—less cost per year added. Other procedures, like heart transplants and surgical implantation of defibrillators (that "shock" you back to life when your heart stops pumping), cost in the range of $75,000 per life year. And some procedures, such as liver transplants, are in the range of $400,000 per life year and are thus clearly less cost effective.

Is it possible to draw the line and say that on the basis of a cost-effectiveness calculation, one should only offer procedures and treatments with a cost-effectiveness ratio below a certain threshold? The Affordable Care Act prohibits us from doing this in the United States (due largely to lobbying efforts of the pharmaceutical industry). But the United Kingdom has a "cost-per-QALY" cut-off: generally new medical advances aren't approved if they cost more than the equivalent of $50,000 per QALY, though this is not a hard-and-fast rule.

Clearly much more work needs to be done to better determine how to measure whether something "works" and then to determine how that should affect what gets paid for. Deciding not to do certain procedures or not to fund certain drugs involves complex ethical, legal, and social issues—which we further discuss in chapter 8.

## Fraud and Abuse

The US Government Accountability Office has estimated that as much as 10 percent of all Medicare and Medicaid billings are fraudulent.[14] Fraud in commercial insurance is about half as common as in Medicare and Medicaid.[15] The top three areas of insurance fraud[16] are as follows:

1. *Billing for unnecessary services or services not performed.* For example, "In Florida, a dermatologist was sentenced to twenty-two years in prison, paid $3.7 million in restitution, forfeited an addition $3.7 million, and paid a $25,000 fine for performing 3,086 medically unnecessary surgeries on 865 Medicare beneficiaries."[17] These charges can be subtle, where is physician sees a patient every two weeks "for needed follow-up" when every six months would have been adequate.
2. *Prescribing unnecessary medications to patients.* The overprescription of opioids we discussed falls into this category.
3. *"Upcoding" for medically unwarranted services or durable-medical-equipment suppliers billing for new equipment when the equipment is used.* "A Roseville, CA, podiatrist submitted over $2.8 million in fraudulent claims for reimbursement. The provider falsely claimed that he performed more expensive procedures which were justified because of illnesses or symptoms that were not present."[18] *Upcoding* is a type of fraud physicians may commit when billing, for example,

for a forty-five-minute outpatient visit when the visit actually only lasted a few minutes; while the payment per patient may differ by only about $100, in a year this could add up to half a million dollars in fraudulent billing for a single physician. [19]

And there are unintended consequences to policing fraud. To discourage upcoding, for example, payers require detailed documentation of what was done at each visit. Documenting this information takes a great deal of time and decreases physician productivity—one of the major complaints physicians have about EHRs. Automated billing—in which a computerized bill is generated in relation to the actual time taken with a patient—will not only eliminate the possibility of upcoding fraud but also restore trust among practitioners, insurance companies, and the government. It would ultimately reduce the administrative cost of proving whether fraud occurred.

## Pricing Failures

In their classic paper "It's the Prices, Stupid . . ."[20] Gerard Anderson and colleagues make the point that the United States continues to be the most expensive place on Earth for medical care. This difference in cost is actually due to high numbers of services offered and performed as well as high prices to perform them. The US system used about 30 percent more services (such as magnetic-resonance imaging) than the British system did, each paid in a fee-for-service system, and spent about 75 percent more per person on higher prices (e.g., in the United States the price of an x-ray would be $175 but only the equivalent of $100 in the United Kingdom).

There are several explanations for this difference. First, in the United States, health-care worker's salaries, medical equipment, and supplies are more expensive than in other countries. Second, the average US hospital stay has more tests and procedures per admission than in other countries. Third, the US health system, due to the large number of ways processes are done, is grossly inefficient. Remember the sheer number of billing clerks required to keep a typical US hospital operating?

If we home in on drug prices, the differences are huge here, too. US spending per person on prescription drugs is more than twice the average spending in other industrialized countries. First, there is no centralized place in the United States for negotiating drug prices. Second, the drug manufacturers say that our higher prices in the United States help support pricing in other parts of the world. Third, drug manufacturers insist that reducing prices would slow innovation—though we believe it's worth having a real conversation about what, exactly, that means. If there are several really important drugs that were discovered and brought to the market with funds that drug makers would not have otherwise had, then maybe we should stop talking about lower drug prices. But drug companies are extremely large and profitable. There's nothing wrong with profit, but when drugs are not affordable and people die, it lends credence to the idea that we need lower-cost drugs. Fourth, Congress has not made addressing drug prices a priority, largely because of pressure from pharma lobbyists.

## Failure of Care Delivery: Safety

"Unsafe" care creates more problems—such as high numbers of infections in surgery, wrong doses of medicine administered, or even the wrong kidney removed in surgery. Looking at medical errors alone, the annual cost is somewhere between $17 and $29 billion every year; more than 250,000 Americans die annually from medical errors: those fatalities are comparable to a fully loaded double-decker Airbus A380 airplane crashing every day of the year. The most common medical errors in the hospital are medication errors (either the incorrect amount or the incorrect drug), too many blood transfusions, falls, pneumonia acquired in the hospital, and infections from intravenous lines.[21]

## Failure of Care Coordination: Readmissions

In 2008, two years before the Affordable Care Act was passed, one in five people admitted to the hospital were readmitted within thirty days of discharge.[22] Each readmission costs an average of $15,000, can prolong a patient's illness, increases their time away from home and family, and exposes them to potential harms such as hospital-acquired infection.

A lack of care coordination—really, a lack of appropriate outpatient follow-up—has been blamed for these readmissions. Most of the reasons for readmission in the first thirty days are associated with a problems with medications, either taking the wrong dose or nonadherence—not taking the medicine correctly or not at all.[23] Depending upon the approach, as many as 82 percent of readmissions can be prevented by a program called Grand-Aides, in which nurse aides augment the work of nurses to assist patients with their at-home care.[24]

It is instructive to consider attempts to reduce patient readmissions made by the Centers for Medicare and Medicaid Services (CMS), the agency that pays for Medicare and Medicaid. When faced with high readmission rates among hospitals receiving Medicare funding, CMS announced in mid-2011 that they would penalize hospitals with high readmission rates for certain diagnoses, such as heart failure. The rate for these readmissions before the penalties was 21.5 percent. The rates began to decrease in 2012 even before the first penalties were levied. Rates continued to decrease through 2013 to 17.8 percent but have not changed appreciably since.[25] In 2018, 80 percent of all hospitals were penalized, with an average penalty of $220,000 total.[26] Yet readmitting hospitals earned $2.8 million for these returning patients' care. Considering that hospitals earned $2.6 million net for those readmissions may help to explain why the readmission rate has not further decreased.

## CHAPTER SUMMARY

- The most well-known study of waste in US health care concludes that about one-third of US health-care dollars are misspent, totaling about $1 trillion annually—a million-million dollars.
- To put this into perspective, removing only a small fraction of waste could cover the uninsured, which would cost between $150 and $200 billion.
- Administrative costs account for the greatest amount of waste—like using more billing clerks than there are beds in a hospital. $250 billion is administrative waste, like using billing clerks; $192 billion is lost to overtreatment, like when physicians order unnecessary tests and procedures; fraud and abuse deplete another $177 billion, most commonly when companies and practitioners bill for a service that wasn't done or was actually cheaper than reported; pricing failures account for another $131 billion in waste, about three times as much per service as in the rest of the world; $128 billion are lost to unsafe practices, with as many patients dying in the United States from medical errors (such as the wrong medication) as would die were a full jumbo jet to crash every day of the year; failures of care coordination waste another $35 billion, when about one in five Medicare patients are readmitted to the hospital, which also carries untold cost in the suffering of the patients and their families.

## Chapter Four

# Myth: Most Medical-Care Dollars Are Spent in the Last Six Months of Life

The United States annually spends 25 percent of the entire $600 billion Medicare budget—that's $150 billion—on patients who die in a calendar year.[1] Medicare spends almost four times as much on the patients who died as was spent on all the other people covered by Medicare, combined. Hospitalization accounts for a huge part of this cost, which accounted for 51 percent of total US medical-care spending in the last year of a patient's life.[2] How do we compare to other countries? As with most other international comparisons, studies show that the United States spends more than any other country. Taiwan, incidentally, spends the least.[3]

In looking at the spending of the last three years of a patient's life, an important observation was made: the cost in the last year of patient life was actually made up of two components: (1) the amount that would have been spent had the patient lived and then (2) the added amount in the last year associated with dying.[4] In the United States, spending in the last three years of a patient's life averaged $155,000 per person—or about $52,000 for each of those years. This is the amount the patient would have spent had they lived. The actual last year of life cost $80,000 per person. This is $28,000 above what would have been spent had the patient not died. Therefore, the spending actually associated with dying is a lot less than a quick look at the numbers might reveal—$28,000, not $80,000. This, to an extent, is good news, as the amount spent dying is less than we previously thought. But the amount spent on chronic disease in those last three years is still huge.

If patients, their families, and their physicians were all satisfied with the processes and with how well this money is spent, it might be worth the enormous cost. But of course, few seem to actually be satisfied.

## THE PROBLEM

So, what's wrong with end-of-life care in the United States?

1.  Family members and patients don't have enough conversations about death and dying. In a recent survey of US adults, more than 70 percent of respondents said that "helping people die without pain" was the most important objective in end-of-life medical care; only 20 percent said that "preventing death and extending life as long as possible" was more important. More than 70 percent of respondents said they'd prefer to die at home, while fewer than 10 percent said they'd prefer to die in a hospital. And patients often don't make those wishes known in a way that ensures they can be carried out. Only a quarter of Americans have written down their end-of-life wishes, and just 11 percent have ever discussed the issue with a doctor. [5]
2.  Health-care providers don't do a good enough job initiating conversations about end-of-life care with their patients and may "push too hard" to keep a patient alive at the end.
3.  We don't know when the last year of life starts.
4.  The topic of death and dying, already difficult, has practically become taboo, thanks to political rhetoric. Former vice presidential candidate Sarah Palin coined the term *death panel* in 2009 when trying to convince voters that proposed health-care legislation would have empowered "bureaucrats" to decide whether terminal patients were deemed worthy of medical care. In reality, no such proposal or law ever existed, and while Palin never won higher office, she did win PolitiFact's Lie of the Year award for her fabrication. [6] But the comment muddied the waters. The damage was done, and stigma around having already difficult conversations intensified. When we talk about end-of-life planning, we aren't talking about cutting patients off from care—or doing anything patients don't want to do. Planning end-of-life care is about respecting people's wishes—and, importantly, giving them the opportunity to express them.

Why does all of this matter? As a nation, we have limited funds to spend on health care. And we're spending a huge portion of it on treating dying people who may not benefit from that treatment and who, in many cases, don't want that treatment anyway. Beware the "helicopter relative"—the previously absent distant relation who, upon learning that their third cousin, once removed, has been hospitalized and is dying, flies in after not seeing them for years, only to insist (presumably to deal with their own guilt over keeping in such lousy contact) that absolutely everything be done for the patient, whatever the cost.

So, what should our possible solutions be for creating quality end-of-life care?

## SOLUTION #1: HEALTH-CARE PROVIDERS NEED TO KNOW THE WISHES OF THE PATIENT

A *living will* is an "advance directive" in which the patient, usually in discussions with the family, decides how much support they want in the event they are dying. These documents can be very specific, including resuscitation instructions (a *do not resuscitate* order, or DNR, means that if the patient's heart stops, efforts to start it again will not be made), intubation instructions (a *do not intubate* order, or DNI, instructs medical staff to not insert a breathing tube), and other directions, such as tube feeding, dialysis, or organ donation. Living wills are legal documents, made to protect the wishes of the patient when they may not be able to speak for themselves. Conversations about death and dying and living wills are important and best had when people are healthy. But only 24 percent of Americans have a living will.[7] Why? The reason given most often is that patients and their families don't even know what a living will is. Or, more likely, by the time the family has decided that the living will applies, the end is too near to do much—maybe only even a few days away.

The Aspen Institute suggests that families bring discussions of advance-care planning into "the fabric of life to be discussed openly and preferably when all members of the family are healthy."[8] All family members should be included in the discussion, or at least be made aware of the decisions, to prevent "Cousin Martha" from swooping in over Joe's deathbed, after a twenty-six-year absence, only to insist that medical staff do everything in their power to keep him alive as long as possible.

Public and private insurance plans should have incentives to encourage patients to develop a plan, particularly at critical points such as the time of enrollment. Large employers should build development of advance-care plans into their employee-benefits programs. And, of course, with all these initiatives there must be mechanisms that allow patients to easily update their plans, especially when they are diagnosed with an illness. Build into all of the above options mechanisms to update the plan at regular intervals—and particularly at the time a person is diagnosed with a serious illness. It is important to note that advance directives can be changed as often as the person wants, right up until the time of death. [9]

Physicians may have difficulty initiating these conversations with their patients. Families may need to gently introduce the topic with their loved one. The Aspen Institute suggests that everyone in the health-care workforce should develop their own advance directives, thereby making it easier to suggest that their patients begin their own planning. [10] The State of New York now requires physicians to discuss advance directives with terminally ill patients. [11]

And patients should ensure their planning has been as complete as possible: A POLST—or a Physician Orders for Life-Sustaining Treatment document—is a doctor's order that only applies in emergency situations. Emergency medical technicians must follow the POLST if it says DNR but will resuscitate an individual no matter what a living will says. Therefore, it is good to have both a POLST and a living will to ensure that your wishes are followed. [12]

Though determining end-of-life care for every patient is important, physicians should not be forced into having these discussions. Nurses, colleagues, community members, and spiritual leaders can also have these discussions with patients. A greater variety of health-care workers should be trained specifically to discuss end-of-life treatment. They need not be professionals. For example, Grand-Aides (specially trained nurse aides) are taught how to facilitate these conversations and have a supervisory nurse to help continue the dialogue. [13] Once the discussions are complete and the patient has expressed their wishes, the DNR order can only be signed by a physician.

## SOLUTION #2: PATIENTS SHOULD COMPLETE A DURABLE POWER OF ATTORNEY FOR HEALTH CARE (DPOA-HC) OR HEALTH-CARE PROXY

The DPOA-HC is a document in which the patient assigns a person to make decisions when the patient is not able to. This is usually a family member, but it could also be a close friend. It is important that the patient go over the living will with the DPOA-HC designee to be certain they will be able to carry out the patient's wishes. For example, if the patient wants very little medical care and their designee disagrees with this decision, then the patient should designate a different DPOA-HC, since in some states, once the patient is no longer competent, the DPOA-HC can countermand prior instructions, including having a DNR taken away.

## SOLUTION #3: WE CAN ALL DO OUR BEST TO IDENTIFY WHEN DEATH IS NEAR

People with progressive chronic illnesses face three distinct phases of illness: (1) "a trajectory with steady progression and usually a clear terminal phase, mostly cancer," (2) "a trajectory (for example, respiratory and heart failure) with gradual decline, punctuated by episodes of acute deterioration and some recovery, with more sudden, seemingly unexpected death," and (3) "a trajectory with prolonged gradual decline (typical of frail elderly people or people with dementia)." As can be seen in cancer, entering a clear terminal phase usually precedes death in a fairly short period. But with heart disease, there can be a number of what appear to be "terminal phases" from which the patient recovers, though never fully. [14]

Understanding the disease trajectory is important, as expectations need to be managed and preparations made for appropriate timing of palliative care and hospice. Providers and researchers should continue to develop better models of trajectory and fit individual patients to those models. Of course, the ideal is to have early old age last as long as possible and late old age last fifteen minutes.

## SOLUTION #4: JOINTLY DECIDE WHEN IT IS APPROPRIATE
## TO ENTER PALLIATIVE CARE OR HOSPICE

The terms *palliative care* and *hospice* are frequently used incorrectly. According to one online medical encyclopedia, the differences are in the goal of the care given:

> The goal of palliative care is to help people with serious illnesses feel better. It prevents or treats symptoms and side effects of disease and treatment. Palliative care also treats emotional, social, practical, and spiritual problems that illnesses can bring up. When the person feels better in these areas, they have an improved quality of life. Palliative care can be given at the same time as treatments meant to cure or treat the disease. Palliative care may be given when the illness is diagnosed, throughout treatment, during follow-up, and at the end of life. Both palliative care and hospice care provide comfort. But palliative care can begin at diagnosis and [be administered] at the same time as treatment. Hospice care begins after treatment of the disease is stopped and when it is clear that the person is not going to survive the illness. Hospice care is usually offered only when the person is expected to live six months or less. [15]

As we've already discussed, physicians also may have difficulty "letting go" and suggesting the proper path for palliative care or hospice. A chaplain once said that the last year of life is more about the doctor's ego than the patient's illness. Physicians sometimes focus on symptom management or treating a disease aggressively rather than face the fact of death.

Similarly, both physicians and nursing homes may believe that a patient who is dying should be transferred to an emergency department for admission to the hospital. There are numerous reasons for this course of action—many of which have to do with the family. Some health-care providers believe this is what families prefer, in part due to some of the issues discussed previously, such as a lack of previous discussions about end-of-life care or even disagreement within the family about what, exactly, the goals of care should be. [16] Many transfer decisions also have to do with malpractice. Cases like a recent $28.5 million judgment against a nursing home for failure to transfer a patient tends to increase the likelihood of transfer. [17]

While nursing homes are not permitted to require a durable power of attorney before accepting a patient, they can strongly suggest that each person admitted have a family member or friend assigned to this role. Discussions between the power of attorney, physicians, and nursing home can practically function as a patient's living will, as they deal in advance with decisions for future care.

## SOLUTION #5: LEARN FROM THE EXTREME ELDERLY

There is a hint that we actually can do better administering end-of-life care: per-person Medicare spending decreased steadily with age among those who died, from a maximum of $42,000 at the age of seventy-three to $18,500 at age one hundred, with the major decrease coming in inpatient hospitalization.[18] Everyone can learn from how the extreme elderly are handled and then apply these concepts to those who die at a younger age. It seems reasonable to discuss with geriatricians and others who care for people of advanced age whether in fact there are intentional discussions that lead to reduced inpatient visits or a reduction in other services.

## SPENDING

Thus far, we have considered ways to make dying better for the patients and their families. This is an important goal itself.

But can we save money in the last year of life? The answer is "As currently practiced, not a lot." Why? For one thing, relatively few people make use of advance directives, DNR, palliative care, and hospice. For another, all of these efforts, even if followed by everyone, are focused on the last month of life—or even less.

1. About 25 percent of people have an advance directive.[19] We would want all people to have advance directives indicating what they want at the end of life. This is the right thing for patients and their families. However, given that these directives currently refer to preferences for treatment administered in the last days to weeks of life, the cost savings to even markedly increasing the number of advance directives will not be great.
2. Even if everyone had a DNR order, the savings would not be highly significant. For example, at Memorial Sloan Kettering, one of the top cancer centers in the world, more than 80 percent of their terminally ill patients have a DNR; yet this does not translate to significant savings.[20]

3. The average duration of palliative care is thirty-four days.[21] As currently practiced, savings from palliative care may not be as large as one might think, because, for example, in cancer treatment, the patient may not require *less* care but care of a different kind. Even if the chemotherapy is refused, the chronic medication and radiation for pain may be just as expensive.

4. The average duration of hospice care is twenty days.[22] Hospice is used most often for patients with advanced cancer, but more and more those with heart, lung, and cognitive failures are using it as well. Hospice can save money.[23] Inpatient hospice saves little, while the major savings are in outpatient hospice, with most savings due to reductions to inpatient admissions and ED visits.[24]

As we discuss end-of-life care, it's worth noting that many of the instructions in advance-care directives really only apply to patients whose death is imminent. Things like feeding tubes, ventilators, and DNR orders are concentrated in the last week or two of life. Perhaps a better goal is to extend palliative care earlier in the course of a patient's treatment.

## THE EXTENDED LIVING WILL

As part of an entry into this program, a whole new consideration—an *extended living will*—could be completed for patients with serious chronic disease with perhaps a two-year time frame in mind.

Discussions could then take place around what a patient and family want as the medical condition begins to worsen. Since the majority of people would likely want to stay out of the hospital (and since their staying out of hospitals also represents major potential for cost reduction), the patient and family could detail what kind of care the patient would want at home. They could also discuss what sorts of symptoms would warrant a trip to the hospital and which symptoms wouldn't.

The extended living will could also detail decisions around types of chemotherapy for cancer or around implantation of a device that helps pump blood for a patient with heart failure or could detail whether the patient wants to be involved in experimental studies. This type and timing of conversation should be more comfortable for a physician to have with the patient, but if not, others could be trained have deal with helping a patient create an extended advance directive.

## IT'S GOING TO HAPPEN

The most important thing to know about death is that it's going to happen. And while it's important for patients to have hope, it's also important to acknowledge the existence of death and prepare for it. The bottom line is that everyone—patients, family members, and doctors—must do more to facilitate end-of-life conversations. "The conversations don't need to be uncomfortable," one ethicist said. "It's just that people don't know how to have them."[25] In fact, it can be incredibly difficult for physicians to say goodbye to a patient they've grown to like, or to admit they are powerless to save them. And some just aren't good at it. Fortunately, others on the health-care team are ready and willing but need to be called upon to step in and help begin one of the most important conversations a person will ever have.

## CHAPTER SUMMARY

- Surveys show that Americans don't want unnecessary, painful, expensive medical care at the end of their lives. Asked what's more important when it comes to end-of-life care, only 20 percent named "preventing death and extending life as long as possible."
- But most don't have the conversations and do the paperwork needed to ensure that they die according to their wishes.
- The result is that we spend a lot of money on futile care in the United States. Twenty-five percent of the entire $600 billion annual Medicare budget is spent on people who died in that year.
- We should work toward achieving five big goals to address this challenge:

  - Increase the percentage of those who have living wills that specifically state what support the patient wants at the end of life.
  - Have patients designate a person to make decisions when they are unable to do so.
  - Improve prediction so that the patient and family know when it's time to prepare for death, entering palliative care and eventually entering hospice without inpatient admissions.
  - Help as many patients as possible to enter appropriate palliative care and hospice.

- Learn from how we manage the extreme elderly; those aged one hundred years or more have fewer inpatient admissions than younger patients.

- We propose that a new *extended living will* be created for patients with chronic conditions who are expected to die within two years, which will provide for medium-term care, bridging the gap created by living wills that really only kick in when a patient starts dying.

*Chapter Five*

# Myth: The United States Consistently Provides High-Quality Medical Care

## WHAT IS QUALITY MEDICAL CARE?

Try this at a dinner party—maybe one that's dull: Ask everyone what they think makes a "good, high-quality doctor." Your friends might say that the doctor is pleasant to talk to, or they're a friend of the family, or it's easy to make an appointment with their office. But here's one quality defining a good doctor that your friends might not have thought about: Does the doctor make you better? You might assume that's a given—after all, we're talking about your *doctor*. But not all doctors are created equal; some are better, and some are "less better" at the critical task of actually diagnosing and treating their patients' medical problems.

We've discussed the cost of medical care, but now it's time to discuss *quality* of care. Surely we wouldn't even want to spend a small amount of money on low-quality medical care. But how exactly can we really define and measure *quality*? Whether we're being treated for cancer, kidney disease, heart attack, or high blood pressure, we want to know whether our physicians are any good. Fortunately, the National Academy of Medicine—a congressionally chartered group of top physicians and others concerned with health and medical care—offers six important aims of high-quality medicine:[1]

- *Patient centeredness.* Does the physician relate well to the patient, consider the patient's wishes and values, and keep the patient informed? This is

the part of quality that our dinner guests referred to above. One measure of this is patient satisfaction, often measured through patient surveys.
- *Timeliness.* Can the patient be seen by the doctor or a nurse practitioner in a timely manner? Or, in other words, will someone see the patient when both the patient and the referring physician want them to be seen?

But in addition to respecting the patient's satisfaction and schedule, there are other dimensions that indicate quality medical care:

- *Effectiveness.* Is the correct treatment done, and is it done correctly? Is the treatment given appropriately to those who need it and not given to those who don't? What are the results of treatment—that is, did the patient get better?
- *Efficiency.* Are resources such as equipment, supplies, and people's time being wasted? Waste is, by definition, bad quality of care, since unneeded tests and treatments are expensive, inconvenient, and possibly even dangerous. One study suggests that 32 percent of sick adults in America have been sent for the same tests within a few days of each other by different health-care professionals.[2] This type of waste qualifies as inefficient since the money can be used in better ways.
- *Equity.* Does everyone have a fair opportunity to receive health care of the same high quality, regardless of the patient's gender, ethnicity, geographic location, and socioeconomic status and whether the patient is insured? In other words, are we treating patients with same diseases the same way no matter, say, their race? Currently we do not. Health disparities exist in the United States. For example, the average Caucasian life expectancy including both genders is seventy-nine years; yet for African Americans it is only 75.6 years.[3] For virtually all forms of cancer, people diagnosed with cancer who have lower incomes suffer higher mortality than do those diagnosed with cancer who have higher incomes.[4] It's a similar story when we consider where patients live: Death rates are higher for people living in rural areas, and the difference is widening. Residents in metropolitan areas have experienced larger mortality reductions over the past four decades than nonmetropolitan residents.[5] But overcrowded areas in cities also experience more deaths: the life expectancy in Harlem in New York City is lower than the life expectancy in Bangladesh.[6] And the data are similar for the uninsured, a topic that we'll discuss in chapters 11, 12, and 13.

- *Safety*. Health professionals are human, and they make mistakes. It has been estimated that ninety-eight thousand patients die in hospitals each year because of medical errors; that's about three hundred people per day.[7] That's not an easy number to conceptualize, so think of it this way: it's the equivalent of a full jumbo jet crashing per day and three times the number of people who die on highways each year. Every day two patients have either the wrong limb amputated or the wrong kidney taken out. Approximately 1–3 percent of all hospital admissions will result in death or harm from injuries, not from the patient's disease but from the medical care itself. The most common reasons for medical errors in the hospital are (1) drug errors (wrong patient, wrong dose), (2) acquired infections in the hospital (blood infection from an IV line, urinary-tract infection, pneumonia, or surgical-wound infection), (3) injury from falls, (4) pressure ulcers, and (5) blood clots.[8]

Why do these medical errors occur? We know that many errors are connected to poor communication among health-care providers as well as to poor communication between the providers and their patients. The patient and family must become a more integral part of the overall care team: all of us should question each other—and ask for help more often—to improve care and help change the processes that currently allow too many avoidable medical injuries.

Health teams have much to learn from the airline industry, which has popularized preflight safety checklists, where team behavior is the norm, and whose copilots are expected to question the pilot. These types of practices have slowly been adopted in operating rooms, where now the surgeon—no less strong willed than any pilot—must check with the anesthesiologist and the nurse to be sure, for example, that the correct side of the body is being operated on (such as in the removal of the correct kidney).

The National Academy of Medicine has defined the six elements of quality medical care. As patients work their way toward understanding true quality care and what would look like to them, they'll need to rank each of the six elements in order of personal importance when choosing a physician or a hospital in which to have a procedure; ideally, every one of these quality indicators is important, but, for example, some patients may be willing to sacrifice timeliness, feeling that waiting an extra month is worth it if it means being seen by a higher-quality specialist.

## GETTING TO QUALITY: HOW ARE
## MEDICAL DECISIONS MADE?

Less than 20 percent of medical decisions are based on "appropriate evidence."[9] Now that we have your attention, let us explain why this is so. Up until about forty years ago, medical decisions were based on clinical experience and information in textbooks or by asking colleagues and experts. For years, quality was indeed in the eye of the practicing physician. High-quality care was taken for granted by both patients and physicians.

This model began to unravel in the early 1970s when research increasingly showed that doctors across the country were treating patients with the same diseases in different ways and that, as we saw above, in more than 80 percent of cases no one really knew what the "best," data-supported treatment was. You might say, "Well, the good doctors knew anyway." Read on.

The "shot heard 'round the world" came in 1991 when the results of the Cardiac Arrhythmia Suppression Trial (CAST) were published.[10] This large clinical trial was designed to shed light on and decrease some of the four hundred thousand sudden deaths in the United States each year due to coronary heart disease. Before the CAST, doctors knew that people often died suddenly after suffering a heart attack. Doctors also knew that the greater the number of extra "premature" heartbeats patients with heart disease had, the more likely they were to die suddenly. In an effort to address this problem, the CAST was designed to see which of the medicines used would decrease the extra beats most effectively and prevent sudden death. Twenty-seven clinical centers around the country enrolled 4,400 patients who had previously had a heart attack and gave them either a placebo (sugar pill) or one of the three drugs used to treat premature heartbeats. The clinical trial was stopped early because it was clear that one group was doing much better than the others. It turns out that the group with the best results was the placebo group. All the actual drugs were making the patients worse! This trial showed us that conventional wisdom in medicine is not always right and that currently held medical assumptions need testing.

Here are a few more myths that we can bust based on new information. Cardiopulmonary resuscitation—CPR—which combines chest compressions with rescue breathing, is no more effective than chest compressions used alone.[11] And breast-cancer survivors, who are often told not to lift weights if they have swollen limbs, actually find their symptoms improve with weight lifting.[12]

In one study, doctors from around the United States examined all articles published over a decade in the highly regarded *New England Journal of Medicine* that examined the "current practice" of physicians. [13] In 40 percent of the studies—that's two in five cases—the current practice either had no benefit at all or was worse than the practice it replaced. Some of the practices found to be harmful possibly affect millions of people daily. For example, very tight control of blood glucose increased mortality in diabetics with hemoglobin A1c levels less than 7.0. [14]

The CAST and other studies demonstrated that there is a need for good evidence to demonstrate what medical practices will actually improve quality care. We also know that some physicians make medical decisions based on traditional teaching, on what "seems to work" based on their experience or their teachers'. Medical training has historically relied on mentor experiences, but unfortunately different people of vastly different experience teach physicians—thus teaching physicians to practice differently on similar patients. The cycle continues when young physicians increasingly learn to rely on their growing "experience" and eventually fail to stay current with new, emerging medical data. In fact, patients of older physicians die more frequently than do patients of younger physicians. "A survey of nearly three quarters of a million patients found that those treated in hospital by a doctor aged sixty or over had a noticeably higher chance of dying within a month than those who saw a doctor younger than forty. For every seventy-seven patients treated by doctors over sixty, one more patient would die." [15]

The take away is this: just because physicians follow a certain medical practice, or just because the practice seems to make sense, doesn't mean the practice is actually right. Data-driven medical care is required.

## PRACTICE GUIDELINES AND EVIDENCE-BASED MEDICINE

Not surprisingly, data show that there is tremendous variation in how patients are treated. For example, in West Virginia a patient is seven times more likely to have a heart procedure than is a patient in San Francisco. But those patients in West Virginians were no sicker. They had no better health results than the San Franciscans, suggesting many had never needed the costly procedures in the first place. There are many similar examples of such overtreatment. One of the main reasons is that many physicians operate on a fee-for-service basis and end up performing too many tests and procedures (for more on this topic, see chapter 3). [16]

To address the variation in care, physicians have been developing "practice guidelines." These are rules of thumb for how to handle the most common illnesses. They are prepared mainly by national societies of physicians such as the American College of Cardiology. Groups of experts produce guidelines indicating, for example, who *definitely* does or does not need a pacemaker or who *probably* does or does not need a pacemaker based on their collective judgment, when the data are less than complete. Patients treated according to the guidelines have better outcomes.[17] In fact, many "quality measures" of physician and hospital performance are determined by how well the practice guidelines are followed.[18]

## TRANSLATING GUIDELINES INTO MEDICAL PRACTICE

As we all know, you can lead a horse to water, but you can't make the horse drink. In medicine we might say that the guidelines can be prepared and circulated, but they may not be followed by physicians. Consider cardiology, for example: one year after the guidelines for good practice were published, 67 percent of cardiologists were following the guidelines, but at five years guideline compliance had decreased to 53 percent. Why wouldn't physicians follow guidelines? Most often because the physician says they don't have time to read them.[19] The other reason that guidelines may not be followed is because the physician does not agree with the guidelines—thinking they "know better."

The most important and valid reason for not following the guidelines is that the guidelines do not apply to a particular patient. In such cases, the decision to not adhere to the guidelines may well be correct. Practice guidelines are created for the "most typical" patient. In some cases, the physician may feel that the guideline is not a good "fit." Perhaps the patient is too old, or too sick, or has too many complicating factors for the guidelines to provide good medical care in their case.

Overall, the probability that physicians will follow practice guidelines is about 50 percent—a disappointing statistic, considering that practice guidelines have been shown to reduce variation and tie medical decision-making to evidence. Ultimately, the guidelines need to improve so that they apply to increasing numbers of patients. An important advance in the use of electronic health records is their increasing inclusion of practice guidelines. Consider one scenario: a physician types "slow heart rate" as a diagnosis into the EHR and the national guidelines for "who needs a pacemaker" are displayed on the screen—since that is a treatment for slow heart rate. But in the not-too-distant future, the EHR will be smart enough to know that particular patient the physician is treating and apply the guidelines appropriate for that specific patient for review by the physician.

## DO WE PRODUCE QUALITY CARE?

So all of these data raise an important question: *do we produce high-quality health care in the United States?* The Agency for Healthcare Research and Quality produces a yearly report card of more than 250 easy-to-understand quality measures of health care trended over a twelve-year period.[20] For example, the AHRQ says one measure of a practice's *access*—meaning whether you can see a provider in a reasonable period—looks at "adults who needed care right away for an illness, who always or sometimes got care as soon as needed." Over the preceding twelve years, this measure stayed exactly the same at 86 percent across the surveyed practices. In fact, 65 percent of the measures of access were unchanged. You might say those are pretty good statistics, but, really, we should have seen at least some improvement in twelve years. Another category the AHRQ measures is *effectiveness*—or how well do things work in the medical practice. They found that "adult patients receiving hip joint replacement due to fracture with adverse events" improved from 16 percent to 11 percent. But "suicide deaths per one hundred thousand population" worsened by 3 percent over the twelve years. Among all measures of effectiveness, only about half improved.

In a broader view of the "whole patient," a recent study looked at whether patients received "quality care" as defined by established national guidelines for thirty acute and chronic conditions. Some of the thirty conditions, for example, included treatment for alcohol dependence, asthma, suspected breast cancer, and heart failure. Overall, only 55 percent of patients received the recommended quality medical care, meaning 45 percent did not.[21] Think back to your school days: in any course you took, earning a 55 percent would have meant getting an F.

In chapter 1 we saw how the United States rates worst among other measured countries for health care—sixteenth out of sixteen countries. If US medical care only manages to provide quality care for 45 percent of patients, we don't need a lot more examples to demonstrate poor quality here.[22]

## DELIVERING HIGH-QUALITY CARE MAY BE EXPENSIVE

Another myth is that high quality of care saves money. Sometimes delivering high-quality care also saves money. For example, if we eliminate waste, we are eliminating services that provide no benefit and also eliminate those costs. However, delivering high-quality care does not always save money. Some estimates suggest that statins—now available over the counter— "would result in 252,359 fewer major coronary events, 41,133 fewer strokes, and 135,299 fewer coronary revascularization procedures over ten years, as well as reduce coronary heart disease– and stroke-related deaths by 68,534 over the same time frame." Avoiding these events "would save more than $10.8 billion in health-care costs while the costs of drug therapy would increase by $28.3 billion. Increased statin utilization is also estimated to cause 3,864 more cases of rhabdomyolysis"—muscle breakdown—"a very rare but severe side effect."[23] Clearly, taking a statin as prescribed—assuming the prescription is correct—is better quality of care, but it is also more expensive.

## VALUE: EASY TO DEFINE
## BUT MORE DIFFICULT TO PRACTICE

We've spent most of this chapter discussing the concept of quality, but it's also important to understand the idea of *value*. Value is expressed as quality divided by cost: Value increases if quality increases whether costs stay the same or decline. But value can also increase even as costs increase so long as quality improves at a higher rate than costs.

It is easy to say that we invest in tests and treatment that produce higher effectiveness for the same or lower cost. One example would be a drug that could extend the life of cancer patients by one year and is the same price as (or cheaper than) existing treatments. Moreover, one might think that if we are truly pursuing "high-value" treatment, we would be happy to spend more dollars on a treatment or test that had an even higher effectiveness but for an increase in cost. An example might be a drug that extends life by two years but is 20 percent more expensive.

But currently it is extremely difficult to find people willing to spend more money on improving much in medical care. We wonder, in fact, whether the definition of *value* should perhaps be redefined as "improving outcomes at the same or lower cost."

We will see in later chapters that *value-based care* is a term that is increasingly being used to distinguish from *volume-based care*. These terms are used most frequently in describing how physicians are paid. A doctor receiving payment based on the number of procedures they perform describes volume-based care, whereas paying doctors based on the quality of care they provide expresses value-based care. As you read those chapters, ask yourself whether any health system will really pay more for value (which they should) or if what they really mean is that they will not reward high volume but will reward higher quality at the same or lower price.

Finally, consider this basic math: We have already established that value is quality divided by costs. AHRQ says our quality of care in the United States is improving only slightly, but we know that the cost of health care in this nation is rising at a rapid rate. That means the value of US health care, at best, is declining.

What does all this have to do with you? Most of you have insurance from an employer, or perhaps you're covered by Medicare. You have largely been isolated from the true cost of care, although you are increasingly paying more out-of-pocket as employers and even Medicare are requiring you to pay more. The average deductible for people with employer-provided health coverage rose from $303 in 2006 to more than $1,200 by 2016 (and it has increased since).[24] If you didn't care about value before, you'd better care about it now. As your personal costs are rising, you're getting less value for your dollar.

## CHAPTER SUMMARY

- Quality in medical care isn't a vague concept. The National Academy of Medicine defines quality as patient centeredness, timeliness, effectiveness, efficiency, equity, and safety.
- National physician associations create practice guidelines that suggest how best to manage patients. Following those guidelines in most cases is thought to contribute to quality medical care, but fewer than 20 percent of the recommendations are based on appropriate evidence. Meanwhile, only about half of physicians adhere to practice guidelines.
- How physicians manage patients, therefore, is quite variable:

- In the 1980s doctors were guessing at which drugs to give patients with irregular heartbeats. It turns out the most effective "drug" was the placebo: patients who received the actual drugs died faster.
- Only 55 percent of patients receive the recommended quality medical care, according to a recent study. Fifty-five percent is a failing grade.

- The good news is the use of electronic medical records will eventually yield higher quality health care, as well as cost savings, as patient-specific guidelines will become available for real-time review by treating physicians.
- Ultimately, we will pay for our medical care based on value, not volume. Value is defined as quality divided by cost. There is a current movement in US medical care away from volume-based care.

*Chapter Six*

# Myth: Consumers Make the Best Decisions about Their Medical Care

Increasingly, consumers must make decisions about their health, including whether they want health insurance and, if they can afford to pay for it, how much they want to pay for it. If their employer offers multiple plans, they will need to decide which one is best for them and their family.

When it comes to actually paying for and receiving medical care, there are more choices to be made. Employees must think about whether their family can afford a particular medical treatment and, if there isn't enough money in the bank, think about what other expenses they'll give up to pay for it. At present the least expensive types of plans are high-deductible health plans—or HDHPs—where the family must themselves pay a certain amount of the medical care—the deductible—before the insurance company begins to pay for the rest of their care. Finally, the family then needs to decide what medical care they want to buy as they are having to pay directly until the deductible amount is reached. For some families, the deductible may be as high as $12,000 per year, essentially making the family pay for all medical expenses unless there is a catastrophic medical event—like an accident or chronic disease—which would be so costly that its payment would exceed the deductible.

If people in the family are uninsured either because an employer doesn't offer insurance or because the family can't afford insurance, it is best to discuss the options. If a family member works, there are people in human-resources departments who can advise, and unemployed persons can call the Medicaid program in their state.

## HOW DO CONSUMERS MAKE DECISIONS?

We consumers buy all kinds of things, and we use all sorts of sources to decide what's worth buying—such as Yelp, *Consumer Reports*, social media, or our friends and family. But when we purchase medical care, we're not as likely to carefully research our decisions as we are when we buy things like clothes or cars. When we shop for a new shirt, we know exactly how much it costs, what it looks like, and how it fits. Best of all, we can return the shirt later if we regret purchasing it. Buying a car is a similar but slightly more challenging process: We don't reliably know how well the car was built or how long it will last—a pretty significant lack of information, considering its cost. It might come with a warranty, but often you can return it to the car dealership within thirty days if you aren't happy. When we're ready to get the car's oil changed, we look for advertisements offering the lowest price. When deciding where to take the car for repairs, we go back to the dealer, take it to a nationally recognized auto mechanic chain, or go where our sister-in-law takes her car. If needed, we ask them to "fix the knock in my engine" and rarely hang around for an explanation of what is wrong.

When it comes to health insurance, we're often in the dark. We spend a lot of money to have it even though we often have no idea whether we'll need it. And when we have a health problem, we often don't know what's covered by our insurance or what's not and why. If we're buying insurance through our employer, they decide how much choice we have in our plans. When we finally get insured, the plan comes with a lot of fine print to read—and good luck doing that, even if you're well versed in health care. We recently looked at a disclaimer on short-term insurance policies that all insurers are required to post. It basically tells the insured, "This is not very good insurance"—but you wouldn't know that from the language. We analyzed the reading level required to understand it: you had to have a graduate degree to make heads or tails of it![1] The only way you find out how quickly the insurance company will actually pay is when they do finally pay—or don't.

The point is that we make purchasing decisions every day about our car, our home, and other things on faith, without complete information, trusting that the result will turn out well. But getting information isn't easy almost in any part of life. Do the repair shops post their results for "fixing unknown engine knocks"? Do car insurers tell you "the percent of claims paid in three days"? We have some tips abut deciding on your medical care.

So how are consumers going to make decisions about their medical care, and how successful will they be? In the end, they may find that the way they make health decisions may be a lot closer to the way they choose shirts, cars, and auto insurance. Consider these following examples.

## Personal Health Care

Earlier in the book, we said that 40 percent of life expectancy comes down to individual behavior. Many people ignore all kinds of information about how smoking and obesity lead to conditions like diabetes, despite the fact that they know better. That behavior is *not* due to a lack of understandable information; it more likely reflects how tough it is to change bad habits. In some cases, people with chronic illness often stop taking their medication, and they fail to show up for appointments. At least half of patients fail to follow their doctor's recommended treatment. When you think of it that way, consumers are not directing their own health care so well, are they?

The public should have *patient-practice guidelines* from their physician to indicate when, generally speaking, a physician visit is needed and why—and the guideline should even say when a visit may *not* be necessary. Of course, the guideline would come with the disclaimer "But of course you can come see me any time" so medical-malpractice lawyers wouldn't have a field day. Doing less, based on good evidence, does not mean withholding appropriate care; quite the contrary, it's practicing good medicine.

Maybe consumers need a nudge. Money seems to drive people, so an increased cigarette tax, a proposed tax on fatty foods or sugary drinks, or increasing insurance premiums on those with clearly self-defeating lifestyles may be required. These steps show clear results. Increased taxes on both cigarettes and alcohol have reduced consumption over the last decades. When the city of Berkeley, California, enacted a 12 percent tax on every twelve-ounce bottle of sugary soda, after a year sales of the drinks fell by 9.6 percent, and bottled water sales increased by 15.6 percent. Shopkeepers did not lose money, however, because the average grocery bill remained the same.[2] In our Texas Medical Center Health Policy Institute survey, we found that consumers largely believe that smokers and heavy drinkers should pay a different level for their health insurance.[3]

Beware apps claiming they will aid your medical care. There are twenty-four million people using more than a thousand apps to help regulate their diabetes. But rarely are data available for app users for longer than six months. Why? People don't use the apps for longer than six months.[4] If you find one that works for you, surely use it. Fortunately, apps will get better and better, but the key is the patient's own behavior, and apps don't yet do a great job of regulating behavior.

## Medical Decisions

Some patients want the doctor to make medical decisions for them. Nevertheless, every patient must be informed of their available choices. They should "direct" their own care when there are a number of treatment options or when personal preferences will make a difference in care. For example, in many cases of prostate cancer and breast cancer, the likelihood of a patient's long-term survival is similar with different medical treatments; however, the after-effects of the different procedures (for example, bladder leaking after prostate surgery) are likely to be viewed differently, and the patient's preference should be the deciding factor in the decision.

The patient must be comfortable with their physician. Much of this comfort is based on personal interaction, but the patients should also have available to them certain facts about the physician—which we'll discuss in greater detail later in this chapter—such as the physician's history of success with certain procedures, including rates of death and complications when compared with other physicians who perform the same work. If a patient requires hospitalization, it is worthwhile to see whether their hospital has earned any ratings of "less than expected"—meaning that the hospital is in the bottom half of providers of that same service—and if so, the patients may want to pay particular attention to those indicators as they relate to their specific illness. If possible, stay away from the bottom-performing half of hospitals.

The choice about insurance benefits can be broken down into five questions:

1. *How much "choice" is important to the patient?* Choosing one's own physician seems to be important to many people. Interestingly, the way doctors are chosen most commonly is to ask one's neighbors or colleagues at work shortly after a move to a new town. This is not always the best way to find a good physician, and there are better ways to do it, which we'll cover below. Then when a doctor is finally found, the patient asks the doctor about other doctors for referral. What seems to matter most is keeping the current physicians that the patient likes. Having access to an outstanding hospital or medical center may also be important to some who already have a history of

illness. Of course, a narrower insurance network may give a patient less flexibility in choosing a particular physician or hospital.

2. *How likely is the patient to need medical care in the next year?* For a twenty-six-year-old, we might think the answer is "Not very likely." But don't forget about pregnancy, automobile accidents, and other unexpected events. Of course, if one is fifty-six, has had a heart attack, and is taking medication, the answer is "More likely." Regardless, insurance coverage of some variety is still essential no matter how old the patient is.

3. *What services should be covered?* This question is likely related to whether anyone in the family has chronic disease, but consumers are also concerned about cost. Is it important to that patient to have mental-health and eye-care services covered? If so, the insurance plan may be more expensive. In many cases, it's necessary to check the fine print to know what's covered and what's not.

4. *How much risk is the patient willing to take?* If one is a "risk-taker" and fairly healthy, then choosing a bare-bones plan—or a *high-deductible health plan*—may be fine, although such basic plans may not cover preventive care, and going without preventive care can cause problems later.

5. *How much money can the patient spend?* Clearly, the more one is willing to spend, the greater choice of benefits, physicians, and hospitals they will have. The amount of the *premium* is usually related to the amount of the *deductible*—the amount the patient pays out of pocket before insurance starts to pay for medical care. As a general rule, the higher the deductible (e.g., $6,000, as opposed to $500), the lower the total premium.

## PATIENTS DO NOT USE QUALITY AND COST DATA WHEN SELECTING HEALTH CARE

Currently, most patients do not use quality or cost data. The Kaiser Family Foundation survey found that one in ten Americans say they saw clinical quality information comparing either hospitals or doctors in the preceding year. But of this low number who viewed the data, the proportion who actually used it to make a choice of provider was even lower—4 percent for hospitals and 6 percent for doctors.[5] Most Medicare beneficiaries did not consider quality information important to them.[6]

Once prospective patients review the data, they have to pay attention to what matters to them. This, in and of itself, requires education. Patients found five physician characteristics to be important:

1. whether the physician accepts the patient's particular insurance (64 percent of patients),
2. office location (37 percent),
3. bedside manner from patient satisfaction surveys (34 percent),
4. doctor education and credentials (31 percent), and
5. office hours (25 percent).

Nowhere in the top fifteen factors that patients considered most important was "The doctor makes me better." In more technical terms, what are the doctor's *outcomes*—like patient death after surgery? "Most beneficiaries had problems interpreting quality information. Many misinterpreted star charts, and while bar charts appear easier to read, many beneficiaries still had trouble interpreting the information on these charts."[7] This is not the fault of the patient. For example, in CMS Hospital Compare, we analyzed the description of the measured "Safe Surgery Checklist" and found that a graduate-school-level education was required to understand it.[8]

This type of comparison shopping for good medical care is increasingly important. We now know that the data on outcomes from hospitals and physicians are very different. As patients are spending their own money—not the insurance company's—they should want to know more. In high-deductible health plans, the insured individual pays the first big chunk of medical expenses—an average of about $6,000—out of pocket, up front. This *consumer-directed health care* requires consumers—who later become patients—to "direct" how best to spend that first $6,000. Sometimes they don't have a choice if they have a serious medical event. But often they do have a choice: Should they spend their money on dental care or a mammogram? What about that annual physical? How will they decide what coverage to select?

The data show that patients do not choose wisely and frequently try to save their own money by cutting back on what is necessary care as well as unnecessary care. According to one study, "patients in the [HDHP] plans were associated with a significant reduction in preventive care . . . and a significant reduction in office visits . . . which in turn led to a reduction in both appropriate and inappropriate care. Furthermore, the plans may be associated with a reduction in appropriate preventive care and medication adherence. Current evidence suggests that HDHPs are associated with lower health care costs as a result of a reduction in the use of health services, including appropriate services."[9]

One possible explanation for these findings is that perhaps patients assume that quality of care is good even if it is not, or they don't want to know one way or another. Imagine getting on a plane and seeing a sign advertising your pilot's "star" rating—three out of five stars. Some people, about to board the plane, may not want to know the rating. This situation needs to change.

## WHAT IS THE GOAL, AND HOW DO WE GET THERE?

In order to make sure that every person receives the quality medical care they deserve, the goal is for the patient to review quality and cost data with the same ease with which they choose other services on the Web, such as when shopping for airlines and hotels. The problem is that medical decisions are complex and the information currently provided is often unnecessarily complicated. For starters, every bit of medical information should be written at a sixth-grade reading level. Patients should complain when written explanations are not understandable.

In the following, we suggest how patients can determine where to get quality medical care: the key is in knowing how, and where, to access important data.

## THE PATIENT'S GUIDE TO QUALITY

### Data on Physicians

Right now, it takes work to find data about quality in medical care. If you want quality information about individual physicians, the data are scarce but are becoming more available every day. Most health plans provide patient-satisfaction data at least for all the doctors as a group and, increasingly, by individual physicians.

If a patient is relatively healthy, "how the doctor relates to them" (patient-centeredness and timeliness) is likely to be extremely important and is something well measured by patient-satisfaction data. For a patient with a brain tumor, however, having a "nice person" as a surgeon may be somewhat important, but knowing the results of patients that surgeon has operated upon should be much more important. The Internet provides a convenient gateway for patients and providers alike when looking for quality measures.

GroupOne has a listing of ten sites offering physician reviews.[10] Often mentioned is Healthgrades,[11] a site that provides comparative-quality information on and consumer ratings for providers. Physician Compare, a site providing information about doctors caring for Medicare patients, has some understandable data like "health promotion and education," but one recent search showed that a medical practice in Houston, Texas, had five stars for "giving antiplatelet blood thinners."[12] Just what percent of the general public can even understand what this means, and even then, do they care whether it garners a five-star rating?

While you are looking for quality medical-care providers, it is best to look at several to get a developed perspective. Here are some interpretations of the data you will find:

- *Board certification.* For example, board certification like internal medicine, and sub-board certification like cardiology, indicates that a physician had to pass a board examination assessing what they know. Many boards and sub-boards require continuing education and examination in order to maintain certification. Therefore, up-to-date board certification is a general indication that a physician has kept up with current practice standards. But board and sub-board certification are not any kind of real indicator of quality. These are helpful only if absent—meaning that if the physician you're reviewing is not certified by the board and applicable sub-board in the specialty, stay away.
- *Education and training.* While individuals who train in "big name" programs may be excellent, so may be those who train in less well-known programs, and so information about education alone may not be very helpful when making a decision about who may or may not be the best doctor.
- *Government disciplinary actions.* Most definitely, if an individual has lost their license to practice, this is a huge red flag, and a patient would want to know that.
- *Malpractice.* Malpractice suits are another red flag, although not as much as they may have been in the past. Most physicians get sued at some point, but the thing to watch out for is multiple suits. The greater the number of claims a doctor has settled, the greater the chances they'll have to pay out another one in the future.[13]

- *Outcomes.* Data on outcomes (e.g., death or complications of an operation) from the care delivered by individual physicians is becoming more commonly available. The best-publicized individual physician-outcome data are in New York State's cardiovascular-surgery database, offered through the New York State Department of Health.[14] Every surgeon in the state who does coronary bypass surgery is included here. But this database illustrates the two major problems with individual physician-outcome data:

  1. The data may not accurately reflect the quality of care provided by physicians who only care for a small number of patients. For example, if a physician only operated on three patients and there was one very sick patient who was a very unusual case and died, the 33 percent mortality may not have the same weight as the same 33 percent mortality rate of a surgeon who has operated in one hundred cases. It isn't likely that 33 percent of this surgeon's cases were "very unusual." Additionally, the mere fact that a surgeon does less than the average number of cases may be a sign that they are not experienced or do not get referrals (for any number of reasons, such as poor results in other procedures that are not listed or even the physician's personality). Low numbers of procedures may have nothing to do with quality and perhaps only be an indication of someone who recently moved to the area and is beginning to accumulate data. In general, physicians who perform procedures (for example, surgeons and interventional cardiologists) have better results the more they do. But it is worth trying to find out from, for example, your primary-care physician why a surgeon has had so few cases.
  2. Data on outcomes (such as death after heart surgery) must be compared only among patients with a similar severity of medical problem. For example, all coronary artery bypass operations are not the same: if a patient has one blocked coronary artery and another has five, the second patient has a more severe problem and carries a higher risk of death from the operation, and therefore the patients' long-term results may be different. It is important to find out—again, try to ask your primary-care physician—whether the data on the individual surgeon are compared for similar severity. If so, the information about the ranking will have the "severity adjusted" or

"risk adjusted." If the data are not severity adjusted, the surgeons who operated on tougher cases and sicker patients may have significantly higher mortality rates. This does not make them "lower quality" physicians; it just may mean they are operating on sicker people.

- *Using the data.* One other problem with this type of data is that they are presented statistically: percent mortality (death) or percent complications (what went badly). Unless you are a statistician, trying to figure out whether one surgeon's statistics are better than another is difficult at best. The best way to approach this is to look for the results for your exact problem for your proposed surgeon and then go to the entire United States as the chosen area for the search; then compare your surgeon with the five best surgeons in the country based on search results. If you have a choice, it is best to select a physician whose ratings are closer to the top but that are at the very least average. It is also worthwhile to know how unusual or complex your medical case is. You should ask your primary-care doctor, "Is my case unusual, or is it like most others?" The more unusual or difficult your case, the more important it would be to choose a physician closer to the top in terms of numbers of cases and results. That surgeon is more likely to be able to deal with unusual and complicated cases. So it is important to look at these types of "report card" data when choosing a physician for a specific procedure. If the data are not on any report card, you can ask those same questions directly of the proposed surgeon. Also use your primary-care physician as an "interpreter" of the data.

## Data on Hospitals

Data for hospitals are much more available than data for physicians. Probably the best overall way to find a good hospital is through US News and World Report, which provides annual national and local rankings of hospitals.[15] A lot of people poke holes in their methodology, but the general ranking seems reasonable.

The Medicare and Medicaid Hospital Compare website compares local hospitals (just enter the zip code) using a simple five-star system. The problem is that if you want to learn a bit more about what is good and not so good about the hospital in question (for example, how they do at certain operations or preventive care), the site's explanations are extremely difficult to understand. But it may be the best comparison we have available—for now.

## AN UPHILL CLIMB FOR PATIENTS AND
## AUTOMOBILE DRIVERS

Patients will increasingly be required to understand what health care is available and how much they should buy. If the data you are considering don't make sense, find someone you trust in the medical field to help you interpret the information. Start with your primary-care provider or that provider's nurse. The Affordable Care Act created the position of "navigator" to help sign people up for medical insurance and help decide which type of coverage to purchase, for example.[16] If you don't understand your insurance options at work, talk to HR or call your insurance company. Often they're pretty good at explaining your benefits. Of course, we think that every bit of medical information directed toward consumers should be written at a sixth-grade reading level, but this is by no means the case. Patients should complain, and not be embarrassed, when written explanations are not understandable.

We recognize that having patients successfully search for and interpret Internet health data may be a long time coming, as we may not want or use data in other areas of our lives either. One website advised car owners that taking an active role in vehicle maintenance was the best way to avoid costly repairs down the line. Sound familiar to the advice to get a flu shot, a mammogram, or visit the dentist? Yet most car owners, the website went on to say, fail to keep up with basic auto care, citing the number of vehicles with low or dirty engine oil or dirty air filters (sound like coronary arteries?). Even with the evidence, how many consumers actually pay attention to that advice about "preventive maintenance" for either their cars or their bodies?

So, in addition to caring for the "informed" consumer, health-care data must be usable for the consumer-patient who has little interest in or motivation to direct their own health care and says to the doctor—as they would say to their mechanic when their car needs an oil change or has transmission trouble—"Fix it; don't tell me how, just *fix* it." At least with our bodies we should take greater care to be informed. We can buy another car, but . . .

## CHAPTER SUMMARY

- Consumers currently make decisions on their medical care in the same way they choose shirts, cars, and auto mechanics.
- Most patients do not use quality or cost data when selecting health-care providers. Only one in ten Americans say they saw clinical-quality infor-

mation comparing either hospitals or doctors in the preceding year, and even fewer used the data to make a choice. The chapter provides help in interpreting which data, such as board certification, are helpful in selecting health-care providers.

- It is not entirely the patient's fault that data are not reliably used, as the data are not always helpful, easy to understand, or consistent.
- But there is plenty of understandable data on how people should take care of themselves—like data showing the effects of smoking and data showing how overeating leads to diabetes—that goes ignored. Borrowing from the fact that higher cigarette prices have shown to curb smoking, consumers need a "nudge" in the form of higher prices for foods and drinks that lead to obesity.
- We provide a patient's guide to quality, which offers important pointers and websites for finding data on physicians and hospitals as well as suggestions how to interpret the data as they are presented.

## Chapter Seven

# Myth: Preventive Care Saves Money

*Preventive care saves money.* Right? Politicians say it. So do many physicians. It seems so obvious, right? Spend money now to prevent a disease, and you can save in the future by not having to shell out to pay to treat the disease. As President Obama promoted the Affordable Care Act—which requires insurance plans to cover preventive care at no cost—he often argued, "We fought for this because it saves lives and it saves money—for families, for businesses, for government, for everybody. That's because it's a lot cheaper to prevent an illness than to treat one."[1]

He's half right. Preventive care absolutely saves lives. That's why we think preventive care is a good thing. But it doesn't save money. The point of this chapter is not to argue the merits of prevention. But unfortunately, all too often, people oversell the benefit of preventive care to include cost savings.[2] For example, in the 2008 presidential race, the websites of all three of the final Democratic candidates—Barack Obama, Hillary Clinton, and John Edwards—touted the financial benefits of preventive care, making variations on the argument that we can pay for the uninsured through the savings we achieve by using more preventive care. Unfortunately, that's just false. "Prevention does not save money," wrote Garson in a February 13, 2008, op-ed in *USA Today*. "Prevention is good medicine, but it is not a fiscal panacea."[3] And much more important, the next day famed health economist Milton Weinstein tried to correct the candidates in a *New England Journal of Medicine* piece. "Our findings suggest that the broad generalizations made by many presidential candidates can be misleading," he wrote. "Although some preventive measures do save money, the vast majority [82 percent from our review] in the health economics literature do not."[4] Preventive care is a good thing. But it's dangerous to focus on prevention as a way to address health-care costs. The costs of health care continue to soar, and to solve that problem, our policy makers must focus on real solutions that we know will actually work. Anything else is a distraction.

But as we'll see in this chapter, the longer we live, the more medical care we use. Willard Gaylin put it best. "There is no such thing," he said, "as preventive medicine ultimately, in that we're all going to die. It means that you prevent a child from dying of a childhood disease, which has a humanitarian purpose but not an economy purpose because he will then live to be a very expensive old man."[5] You didn't see anyone in the 2016 presidential election making the same mistake as in 2008.

As we have continued to refine our understanding of what it would take to reform our health-care system, three preventive strategies consistently emerge as potential cost-savers. In the following we explore whether they are, or not.

## 1. CORPORATE WELLNESS PROGRAMS

There's a good chance you've had an employer at some point offer you a free or discounted gym membership. Surely, employers thought, giving employees gym memberships, having them complete biometric screening, and then having them attempt lifestyle changes related to findings from the screening such as dieting, exercising, and smoking cessation must save money, right? No. That's *another* myth.

A recent article *Harvard Business Review* is aptly titled "Corporate Wellness Programs Lose Money."[6] After all the costs and benefits of these programs are added up, they are found to lose about fifty cents per employee per month. Okay, so maybe these programs don't save money, but they're great for morale, right? The employees know the employer "cares about them." Well, not exactly. In one famous case, Penn State University generated national news for imposing a $100 penalty on employees who declined to fill out a questionnaire of health information that contained what many considered intrusive queries, including questions about employees' financial situation and whether they intended to become pregnant.[7] Penn State's wellness program became every human resources director's worst nightmare when the national news reported that "Penn State struck a chord with millions of employees everywhere who have started posting similar stories of invasion of privacy, misinterpreted lab values, and unnecessary test expenses. As these employees expressed it, wellness had become another tool to force them into toeing the corporate line."[8]

But didn't the program at least identify disease early? The *Harvard Business Review* did the math: "Their forty-three thousand covered lives probably incurred a total of only about one hundred wellness-sensitive medical inpatient events, like heart attacks, of which a few might have taken place in people who were not previously diagnosed and were therefore at least theoretically avoidable, saving the tiniest fraction of their healthcare spending."[9] That's a fancy way of saying "no."

For many, the medical costs of obesity (diabetes, heart disease) and smoking (cancer, emphysema) occur years later.[10] The obese young or even middle-aged person does not usually have significant medical expenses (unless they are approaching *morbid obesity*, which is one hundred pounds over ideal weight), and therefore a company might only see savings for those employees who keep their jobs for a long time. In today's world, that isn't likely, as employees change jobs frequently.

The longstanding myth that prevention saves money has led to the rise of a corporate wellness industry that, at best, has neutral results, while at worst it breeds suspicion, resentment, and poor morale among employees, as well as losing money.

## 2. PREVENTION OF CARDIOVASCULAR DISEASE

### Hypertension Screening and Treatment

Consider the case of high blood pressure: Patients with high blood pressure have higher rates of stroke and coronary heart disease and lower life expectancy. In preventing high blood pressure, the costs involved include, first of all, screening the entire population, a very expensive undertaking. Then we would need physician follow-up. Approximately forty-three million Americans have high blood pressure; twenty-three million are treated, and only about half of them have controlled the condition—a quarter of the total.

Once diagnosed, treating a patient with high blood pressure requires physician visits, lab tests, and medications. But there are other costs as well, such as inadequate blood pressure control causing more doctor visits and new medication, not complying with therapy, and lack of follow-up care. So in evaluating the costs of treating high blood pressure we would have to add up the costs of general screening of the population, the treatment costs of those identified as having high blood pressure, and also the costs of those who were hypertensive but never knew it and became ill as a result of their condition. In one study, using a model, it was estimated that $30 billion were spent on treating hypertension, of which about a third—$7 billion—went to paying for medications.[11]

In an estimate of the savings produced by controlling blood pressure, of those with severe hypertension

- 44 percent will not have a stroke,
- 21 percent will not have a heart attack,
- 10 percent will not get kidney disease, and
- 5 percent will not go blind.[12]

The economics of treating high blood pressure depend on how high the blood pressure is and what the risk is of having a stroke or a heart attack. Overall, the cost of prevention is about three to four times the cost of the diseases caused by high blood pressure.[13]

But that's not all. In that period of time, patients will contract another disease, and it is likely that the disease they die from will be as expensive as the one prevented. If we treated your hypertension, we might have saved money by potentially preventing you from having a stroke that would require costly medical care. But that doesn't mean you'd live disease-free the rest of your life. Instead, you might suffer from cancer—another expensive condition. From an economic standpoint, prevention saves the cost of dying from diseases related to hypertension but ultimately contributes to more costs over time: the cost of prevention of hypertension *plus* the cost of dying from a disease not related to hypertension.

But, you might say, what about the economic value of living longer? Shouldn't we save money because those extra years of increased health are productive and an opportunity to earn money? But the ten years of life one gains over those with high blood pressure are years that mostly occur when people are retired and receiving Social Security and Medicare payouts. Although a person is extremely important to their family as a grandparent and to life-long friends, they aren't putting new money into the economy postretirement.

This type of calculation weighing the economic benefits and costs of prevention to society seems very cynical, but it emphasizes our earlier point.

We control diseases like hypertension to add years of life and to promote health, as we should—*not* to save money. In the future, as people remain healthier right up to death, prevention may well save the overall system money. But that's not what's happening now.

## 3. SMOKING

A well-done study looked at the cost of smokers to employers and found that the highest costs were related to missed work—not medical care. The greatest expense was smoking breaks, estimated at eight to thirty minutes per day of lost work time, which averaged a cost of more than $3,000 per employee, per year. Absenteeism (about two days per year) and *presenteeism*—or the lack of productivity due to smoking—followed as the second and third greatest financial losses smoking workers incurred for their employers. "Although cigarettes satisfy a smoker's need for nicotine, the effect wears off quickly," the researchers write. "Within thirty minutes after finishing the last inhalation, the smoker may already be beginning to feel symptoms of both physical and psychological withdrawal. Much of what smokers perceive as the relaxing and clarifying effect of nicotine is actually relief from their acute withdrawal symptoms."[14]

The total workplace expense of smokers was calculated to be more than $4,000 per employee, per year, about double any medical expense. In these cases, clearly, smoking-prevention programs saved the companies money. However, the smokers died earlier, providing a "death benefit" (the article's words) to their employers, who with the death of the employee had to pay lower pension and health-care expenses, which cost an average of more than $10,000 every year for male employees.[15] In this case, smoking saved employers money since the retiree benefits they provided were only paid to patients when they were alive, and the smokers died sooner.

In the 1990s, certain documents were leaked from cigarette companies, showing the companies had long been aware that people become addicted to tobacco. Many states filed suit against the tobacco companies, arguing that smoking causes health problems resulting in significant costs for public-health systems.[16] In 1998, forty-six states settled with four tobacco companies. The Master Settlement Agreement, as it became known, required tobacco companies to pay states annually for health-care costs associated with smoking (tobacco companies agreed to pay at least $206 billion over the first twenty-five years). The Master Settlement Agreement "forbids participating cigarette manufacturers from directly or indirectly targeting youth[,] imposes significant . . . restrictions on advertising, marketing and promotional programs . . . [,] and bans . . . transit advertising, most forms of outdoor advertising, . . . [and] product placement in media."[17]

Note that the Master Settlement Agreement was written in 1998. A paper published fourteen years later could have potentially reversed the agreement: This 2012 study demonstrated that smoking actually saves money for the US government, as the time a smoker is covered by Medicare is less than the time of coverage for nonsmokers, since the smoker dies earlier. The study, reported in the *New England Journal of Medicine* modeled the thirty-year effects on the federal budget of an increase today in the federal cigarette tax of fifty cents per pack (correcting for inflation). The current tax is $1.01. Currently, cigarette smoking causes shorter lives due to cancer and other lung and heart disease. The increase in cigarette tax modeled in the paper would result in less federal spending on Medicare, and the study found that by 2021 almost 1.4 million adults would be nonsmokers because of the policy and that those numbers would continue to grow. The reduction in smoking would cause increased longevity and an increase in health-care costs related to living longer. The higher cigarette taxes would bring in more revenue but would not balance the increase in costs from living longer without smoking-related illness.[18]

## A COUPLE OF FINAL THOUGHTS

First of all, there's certain basic math at play when we think about the role of prevention in medicine. Health-care costs are growing at a much faster rate than inflation—at a current rate of 3.4 percent per year, compared with 2 percent per year for general inflation.[19] For example, a coronary bypass operation is priced at $150,000 today;[20] ten years from now it might be priced at $250,000. But future medical care will be more expensive still: the longer we live, the more expensive our health care gets relative to the consumer price index, and in ten years, the same treatment will be 16 percent higher than it is now.

The second important thought we wish to close this discussion with is that 80 percent of the strategies used to prevent disease are good at keeping a patient alive, but because the patient lives longer, their health care is increasingly expensive. It's important that we concentrate on the 80 percent of preventive care that currently does not save money, largely because people live longer and spend plenty of money. If we want prevention to save money, we will have to devote serious research money to keeping people alive and without symptoms from chronic disease so that ideally early old age lasts as long as possible and late old age is delayed until the final minutes of life.

Remember, though, prevention is not about saving money. We are all here to have as long and happy lives as we can. Prevention helps us to get there.

We end with accolades for a good man: Business owner Bill Crutchfield created an incentive plan to help every one of his employees stay healthy. He supports this wellness program for his workers not because it saves him a lot of money but because it's the right thing to do.[21]

## CHAPTER SUMMARY

- Prevention in health care is good and something we should strive for—but not because it saves money.
- Curiously, politicians and others often tout the myth that preventive care saves money, even though this is only the case about 20 percent of the time.
- Why doesn't preventive care save money? The longer you live, the more expensive you become.

  - A well-done study calculated the long-term effects of a fifty-cent increase in the cigarette tax. In the long run, the less people smoke, the longer they live, and the greater the cost is to paying for their health care.
  - Most employee-wellness programs cost a lot of money, but they rarely actually identify disease early or change habits. Many of these programs may actually hurt employee morale.

- The three final Democratic presidential candidates in 2008 all said their health-care plans would pay for the uninsured with savings found from prevention. When it was widely pointed out that a great percentage of prevention costs and doesn't save money, each candidate removed the claim from their website: the money simply is not there.
- Remember, prevention is good, even though it's expensive.

*Chapter Eight*

# Myth: The United States Will Not Ration Medical Care

Dr. Hagop Kantarjian, chair of the Leukemia Department at the University of Texas MD Anderson Cancer Center, a highly respected cancer center, has spoken about rationing in health care.[1] Rice University's Baker Institute for Public Policy has found that between 2000 and 2015, new cancer drugs rose in cost per patient from less than $10,000 to about $145,000.[2] Kantarjian has seen the impact of those price hikes firsthand. He estimates that in 2018 about 40 percent of his leukemia patients were receiving less-than-optimal care because they couldn't afford the leukemia drugs that would give them the best chance of fighting their cancer. It was a stunning admission from a key leader at one of the world's most respected health-care providers. Kantarjian didn't mince words when he explained what happens to those patients: "They just disappear and don't take the drug, and they die . . . That's the reality of my clinic—every day."[3]

The situation facing Kantarjian's patients is a clear example of medical *rationing*, a term that's become a "third rail" in some policy—and especially political—discussions about American health care: "Touch it, and you are dead," Garson wrote not long ago with colleague Carolyn Engelhard in an issue of *Governing* magazine. "Rationing is the opposite of the American dream: you know, that dream in which we can all have everything, like living forever (or, at least to well over one hundred) with good health and white teeth until the day we die. Mix that with a generation of us 'Baby Boomers' used to having what we want when we want it."[4] But situations like the one Kantarjian described show that the dream might not be so attainable after all.

Sure, we theoretically have access to the best cancer drugs, but that doesn't necessarily mean you or your family can actually get them: those drugs have been "rationed"—or, put more bluntly, saved for families who can afford them.

Rationing angers people frustrated that the American dream may be out of their grasp and frightened that they may not be able to get they help they want to stay alive as long as possible. Rationing means we *cannot* all have it all. There has been some debate about whether Americans could be subject to rationing in the future were the federal government to play a greater role in providing health care. But don't let anyone tell you differently: we already *have* rationing here in the United States.

There are two types of rationing: *Explicit* rationing means you've been expressly told, "You can't have that." As we see above, explicit rationing occurs in determining who gets expensive cancer drugs. There's also much more subtle *implicit* rationing, where access to care—whether all care or certain types of care—is limited indirectly by factors such as the price of care or the distance required for people to travel to get to that care.

Why does all of this matter? Rationing is an important concept that can be spun in multiple ways. From a positive perspective, rationing allows for a more efficient allocation of limited resources. Put more plainly, we can help improve the health of more people if we limit spending on futile or ineffective health care and instead direct our money toward cost-effective treatments that work. But from a negative perspective, rationing can be seen as a way to deny care for the sick in an attempt to preserve profits. Which view is right? As you'll read in this chapter, it's not so black and white.

## EARLY ATTEMPTS AT "EXPLICIT" RATIONING IN THE UNITED STATES

### A New Machine to Treat Kidney Disease

Since government-supported health care was first introduced in the United States in the 1940s, there have been several attempts to ration health care. Let's go back to the early 1960s when a new machine that provided *dialysis* for people with kidney failure was just becoming available. These machines took people who were otherwise certain to die and kept them alive by removing excess fluids and toxins from the blood when the kidneys no longer could. But the number of dialysis machines was severely limited, and dialysis was extremely costly. Decisions had to be made—who would be put on the machine and live, and who would be denied the treatment and die. Committees were formed of doctors, nurses, clergy, and others to help decide who should receive dialysis. They reviewed the "worthiness" of individuals to receive the service. While these committees tried, they became increasingly frustrated, and many simply threw up their hands and said they could not decide.

So the federal government stepped in, and by 1970 Congress approved dialysis for all those with kidney failure and decided to pay for it through a relatively new health-care program called "Medicare."[5] Treatment for chronic kidney disease—for patients of any age—was added to Medicare coverage largely because America was unable to ration health care. By the 1990s, the Chronic Renal Disease Program used 5 percent of Medicare funds for less than 0.5 percent of Medicare's population. Today it accounts for 9 percent of Medicare payments. Collectively, as a country, we've decided to not deny these patients this life-saving care, despite the cost. Of course, this isn't a negative commentary about the worthiness of treating kidney disease but only a fact about our inability to make tough decisions regarding the availability of medical care, particularly when a new service is offered, the need is great, and patients demand it.

## The Oregon Rationing Experiment: A Model for the Future?

A quarter century ago, the public attempted once again to ration health care when the state of Oregon initiated its Medicaid program in 1994. Years prior, Oregon officials had already determined that many of their citizens were going without needed medical care because they were uninsured and not eligible for Medicaid. They also knew that it would be impossible to provide every medical service for every uninsured person in the state, so Oregon policy makers proposed a plan that offered health coverage to those without insurance by enrolling them in a revised Medicaid program. The only way to pay for this new group of people was to limit—or ration—care. The Oregon Health Services Commission was formed to create a list of approximately seven hundred medical conditions and their treatments. The list categorized the medical services as *essential services* that prevented death with full recovery (for example, appendectomy), as *very important services* that improved quality of life (for example, migraine headache treatments), as *services valuable to certain individuals* (for example, infertility services), or, finally, as treatments that had only *minimal effect* (for example, end-stage cancer treatments that were unlikely to significantly prolong life). Oregon Medicaid was then going to start off the year paying for treatments beginning at the top of the list, covering essential services (such as the appendectomy) and continuing to fund medical care on down the list until the state Medicaid money ran out at the end of each year.[6]

We have a lot to learn from the decisions and choices that went into this Oregon rationing experiment. First of all, officials involved couldn't agree on how to rank the conditions and services. They began using straightforward cost-effectiveness analysis (a process we discussed in chapter 3), but they could not agree on what should be considered *essential* versus *very important*. To "fix" the problem, they used focus groups made up of members of the general public to decide which services would be on the list. Interestingly, this selection process caused problems, because many of the members of the focus groups were health-care practitioners who often thought that the most important conditions to pay for were those most related to their area of practice.[7]

Consensus at town halls was difficult to find, and the commission produced the final list by doing what it thought was right. Number one on the prioritized list were conditions classified as *acute fatal*, like appendicitis, and it ended with number seventeen, *treatment causes little improvement in quality of life.*[8]

However, in the summer of 1992, when the Oregon plan (with its list of prioritized covered benefits) was submitted to the federal government for approval, it was rejected on the grounds that it discriminated against people with disabilities and violated the federal Americans with Disabilities Act.[9] "The Oregon Medicaid proposal for rationing services, which used both cost-effectiveness analysis and a quality-of-life-outcome measure to prioritize treatments . . . systematically disadvantaged people with preexisting disabilities."[10] In short, the rankings did not take into account the relatively high quality of life actually experienced by those with disabilities. The rankings were changed, and two years later, in 1994, the plan was approved.

But all was not well. "Shortly after the Oregon program began, the system began to unravel. This failure resulted, in part, from the federal government requiring coverage of almost all services for certain groups (such as those with disabilities), as well as practitioners figuring how to get around the 'rules' to ensure their patients got the treatments they recommended. As a result, Oregon's rationing system covered about the same number of people as before the system was started and, in turn, spent about the same amount."[11] But what Oregon did was demonstrate some benefits—and many pitfalls—of explicit rationing in the United States. The lesson of the Oregon "experiment" is that true rationing is easier in theory than in practice, given the tendency of policy makers, patients, and physicians to each favor a system that works only for them.

While Americans haven't made complete peace with explicit attempts to ration health care, *implicit* rationing is happening already, in several ways, as we'll discuss in the following.

## IMPLICIT RATIONING IN THE UNITED STATES

### Lack of Access

The United States does ration medical care—even though the rationing going on today might not seem as obvious as the rationing attempts in Oregon. The ultimate rationing tools in the United States are lack of health-insurance coverage and lack of access to needed medical care. As we discussed in chapter 1, *coverage* is defined as having health insurance, whether paid for by the employer, the government (Medicare, Medicaid, state or county hospital), or the individual. We ration health care in this country by allowing tens of millions of people to go without any insurance coverage, and let us not forget the many insured people who find their coverage inadequate.

The uninsured get about half the amount of care of the insured, which is definitely a form of rationing as well.[12] It is a misconception that the government provides coverage for all low-income people. Coverage is limited most obviously in the Medicaid program, where in some states such as Texas as many as 26 percent of children who are eligible for Medicaid and CHIP do not sign up.[13] The reasons for this "lack of access" to health insurance through the Medicaid program may be because applicants—or their parents—are required to appear in person but have no transportation, are concerned that a member of their family could get deported, do not have the appropriate documentation to prove how poor they are, or may be unable to complete a complex application form.[14]

### Experimental Treatment

Consider the following statement, which is found in many health-insurance plans: "Insurance companies do not pay for experimental treatment." On the surface, this exclusion seems reasonable. If a company wants to draw a line to limit services in an attempt to hold down costs, this is a place to start. When resources are scarce, it would only make sense that they want to avoid paying for unproven treatments. But we should ask: Whose definition of "experimental" should we use? In many cases, a treatment is deemed experimental by an insurance company's medical director who has personally decided that there is insufficient credible evidence that the treatment works. There is nothing necessarily wrong with that kind of determination as long as the decision is truly based on evidence and is not arbitrary and as long as other medical directors across the country use similar criteria to decide what is experimental. Unfortunately, that is not always the case.

Interpretations can vary about what therapies are medically necessary and when new treatments should be reclassified from "experimental" to "accepted medical practice." As a result, the mix of services actually covered varies greatly from insurer to insurer. For example, there are differences among eight insurance-plan formularies in Minnesota in what is covered, largely based on which drugs are most expensive. One might say that the most restrictive plan is rationing more than the least restrictive plan.[15]

## Self-Rationing

Finally, another rationing strategy used by insurance companies and employers is requiring patients to ration themselves. This type of self-rationing plays out in a significant way with high-deductible health plans, which are becoming increasingly common. Patients now are forced to decide how much health care they should utilize based on their ability—or lack of ability—to pay for it. The US Internal Revenue Service defines a high-deductible health plan as any plan with a deductible of at least $1,350 for an individual or $2,700 for a family.[16] In reality, this number can be $5,000 or more. That means patients effectively have to spend thousands of dollars before insurance really kicks in. This forces them to make tough choices: *Do I really need that surgery? Can I get by without that expensive medication?* As we saw in chapter 6, consumers may not always make the best decisions about their own rationing. It is essential that consumers become more fully informed about all areas of medicine, surely including insurance, with a variety of educational strategies developed to assist the broadest range of people.

## EXPLICIT RATIONING IN THE UNITED KINGDOM

We are not alone; every other country in the world rations.

The United Kingdom has the most public, widespread system for explicit rationing. Its National Institute for Health and Care Excellence—or NICE—was originally set up in 1999 "to reduce variation in the availability and quality of [National Health Service] treatments and care."[17] For example, in certain locations in the United Kingdom, certain drugs were not available, which meant that outcomes of diseases like cancer could be region-dependent. NICE is independent of government, publishing guidelines on medicines, treatments, procedures, and clinical practice, among other areas.[18]

The drugs that NICE considers have already been licensed and deemed safe by the European Medicines Agency. The question NICE tries to answer when determining whether to cover their cost is whether those drugs deliver value for money. The organization's evaluations are delivered mostly in terms of cost effectiveness—a ratio of the cost of the medicine to the life years gained as a result of receiving the medicine (see chapter 3 for an in-depth discussion). The number is usually reported as the cost per *quality-adjusted life year*—or QALY—which takes into account whether the years of added life are somewhat reduced in quality—such as during cancer chemotherapy. The threshold NICE uses is equivalent to about $50,000 per QALY. This number is somewhat arbitrary and is arrived at in a somewhat circular way, by deciding that "most treatments that are in common use" are in this range. The most important thing to know is that if a drug costs more than $50,000 for every year of life it adds to a patient, NICE is less likely to look at it favorably, and the drug is therefore less likely to be paid for by the National Health Service. This is not a firm limit, however. For truly innovative treatments, NICE allows higher prices. NICE also may require pharmaceutical manufacturers to share in the cost of some medicines until data demonstrating wide effectiveness are developed.

"The [UK] NHS Constitution states that patients have the right to drugs and treatments that have been recommended by NICE."[19] If a patient's doctor believes the drugs to be clinically appropriate, the NHS must pay for them. This provision has created a great deal of disagreement from a number of quarters, including patients who want access to drugs, pharmaceutical companies wanting higher prices, and the parts of the NHS that have to pay for the drugs—and thus want lower drug prices and fewer drugs approved.

The constitutional provision has thus far resulted in an amazingly high number of drugs being approved—approximately 85 percent.

For example, in 2009 NICE gave a preliminary recommendation that the NHS should not offer the drug Sutent for advanced kidney cancer. Making this particular decision might have seemed clear-cut, as Sutent costs more than $50,000 per QALY while only offering about six months extra life. However, as the *New York Times* writes, "the British media leapt on the theme of penny-pinching bureaucrats sentencing sick people to death." The story gained traction in the United States, largely because we were embroiled in our own health-care debate in the run-up to passage of the Affordable Care Act. The story of rationing run amok was seen as a cautionary tale in some political circles here. In the wake of the media coverage, NICE eventually recommended that NHS pay for Sutent.[20]

In summary, at present, the forces against public explicit rationing are alive and well in the United Kingdom.

Overall, it seems most likely that the best way to explicitly ration is to get patients to decide for themselves: There is considerable evidence that patients who are fully informed about their medical choices tend to make more conservative decisions about their treatment than doctors—that is, they want less. This has been well demonstrated in men with prostate cancer who have been counseled by physicians other than their treating doctor, using a video explaining their medical-care choices in a "neutral" way, not favoring one or the other; this group is more likely to choose to wait rather than have an operation.[21] As we saw in chapter 4, this is also the case in many patients and families facing end-of-life decisions: patients want less medical care than many doctors want to provide.

## IMPLICIT RATIONING IN OTHER COUNTRIES

We hear that "All countries have universal coverage"—at least, all besides the United States. But it is only true in the sense that each person has a card indicating that they have "government health insurance." No country guarantees universal access to care. The only guarantee is that each person has that insurance card providing access to *some* care. Virtually every country other than ours has an overall budget for health. This limited funding pays, for example, a certain amount to each hospital each year. The hospital has enough supplies for a specific number of operations. It becomes the problem of the hospital and physicians to decide the types and number of procedures that can be performed each year within the budget. Since there are generally more procedures required than money available, less seriously ill patients are "delayed until next year" and may be put on waiting lists. Clearly, some life-saving procedures such as cancer surgery and coronary artery bypass surgery cannot wait—and may be done relatively quickly or receive high priority on the waiting list—whereas other, more elective procedures, such as hip replacement, are moved further down the list. While it is true that some patients die "while waiting on the waiting list," it is more common that patients live but have a lower quality of life while waiting for their procedures.

The presence or length of a waiting list is dependent upon the overall health budget, the hospital's budget, the expense of each procedure, and who ultimately is thought to need the service. Any of these variables can be changed to eliminate waiting lists if a country so desires—including, for example, France's willingness to call this budget a "health-expenditure target" and routinely exceed it.[22] As we will see in chapter 17, Americans are particularly unwilling to wait for medical care, whereas patients in Canada and the United Kingdom are more willing to wait as part of their sociology.

According to Ashish Jha, writing for the Harvard School of Public Health, what that government insurance buys varies across different countries. For example,

> A few years ago, China launched a major health reform with the goal of getting to universal coverage. They got close and nearly every citizen now has health insurance that covers at least part of the costs of their care. The insurance has substantial co-pays and doesn't cover more expensive drugs and tests. What does this mean for a hospital like HDPH? About 40% of their revenues came from insurance. And, despite being a government hospital, only about 5% of revenues came from the government. The rest? From the patients themselves. This revenue mix is supposedly pretty typical of county and secondary hospitals across the nation. Out of pocket spending remains substantial, despite universal health insurance. In fact, in absolute dollar terms, patients are paying about as much out of pocket now as they were before social insurance kicked in.[23]

The world over, there is implicit rationing of health care by ability to pay.

# WHERE DOES THE UNITED STATES GO FROM HERE?

## Rationing in Theory

Everyone can't have everything. We don't have the money. The cost of health care is too high for individuals, for employers, and for the country at large.

But we don't want to ration medical care for several reasons: (1) For most of us, the actual expense of medical care doesn't hit us—it hits the insurers. Therefore, it is easy for us to say that everyone should have everything. (2) We hate the idea that medical rationing could happen to us when we—or our families—are not prepared to bear the fallout. (3) We dislike rationing so much that we bring lawsuits at even the mention of "the R word."

Let's think broadly for a minute about how we could approach "doing less." The place to start, of course, is to deal with waste. If *waste* is defined as something that does no good but has a cost, it is easy to figure out what's waste in the medical system and what isn't. But what if something does "a little bit of good"? Should we nonetheless try to see how we might approach making decisions even the way Oregon did? We must consider cost. Dr. John Eisenberg, one of the fathers of health economics, was ahead of his time when he said in 1989 that "to suggest that medical decision making can be divorced from consideration of cost denigrates the complexity of patient care . . . Almost all clinicians would agree that, at some point, the extra money spent on tiny improvements in clinical outcomes is not worthwhile and represents inappropriate practice."[24]

We must also consider how much good the treatment will provide. These choices must be made as ethically as possible. Each of us needs to carefully create a framework for ethical decision-making to us when considering medical decisions—whether those decisions are being made concerning our own health care or we're operating as members of a concerned public wanting input into the best medical decision-making possible. Surely there are myriad approaches to ethical medical decision-making, but Dr. Ezekiel Emanuel wrote one of the best treatises on the topic in his 2009 article "Principles for Allocation of Scarce Medical Interventions."[25] He discussed ethical principles that should be considered and then how to combine them into a system for decision-making. Think how you would behave were you in charge of making decisions for your town in rural Alaska after an avalanche had hit and only limited resources were available, with no more coming for several months. We outline for you in some detail a system for rationing that does consider a number of important issues and takes the notion of allocating medical care from a hazy idea to something more actionable and useful as we all begin to process the fact that we all can't have it all.

To borrow from Emanuel and colleagues,[26] when deciding who gets medical treatment, the following principles can be helpful—though each one may not apply to every case:

1. *Treating people equally.* This means that everyone has the same chance of being chosen. Think of it like setting up a lottery for medical care: everyone has an equal chance of winning.
2. *Favoring the worst off.* There are any number of ways to do this—you could choose to treat the sickest first, for example.
3. *Maximizing total benefits.* In other words, work to either save the greatest number of people today or else save the people who could live the longest (for example, children, who have the most number of years to live if they are healthy).
4. *Promoting and rewarding usefulness to society.* In recognizing future usefulness, we might choose to provide medical treatment to physicians who would then be well enough to treat sick people in the future, or we could recognize past value, such as providing the president of the United States or a major-league baseball player or a veteran with medical care.[27]

Emanuel makes the point that none of these criteria for care by itself is sufficient and proposes what he calls a new "Complete Lives System," which considers a number of variables:

1. Consider the person's age, but with modifications: "Prioritize adolescents and young adults over infants. Adolescents have received substantial education and parental care, investments that will be wasted without a complete life. Infants, by contrast, have not yet received these investments . . . Individuals aged between roughly fifteen and forty years get the most substantial chance."[28] Those over sixty are still ranked higher than babies up to about three years of age, using the above reasoning.
2. Consider their prognosis—or how many years they are expected to live.

3. When comparing two people, if age and prognosis are roughly equivalent, use a lottery, and consider future usefulness in emergencies—such as whether an individual is a physician or nurse.

4. Finally, include a few people very highly valued to the population.

Emanuel and his coauthors make the point that just deciding to treat the sickest first and be done with it doesn't work, because it is so often gamed in allocation schemes—as with the United Network for Organ Sharing transplant-scoring system, in which physicians may score their own patient as sicker than they really are in order to move them up in priority.

## Rationing in Practice

How will we deal with the ever-increasing availability of new diagnostic tests and treatments that are increasingly expensive? Garson and Engelhard "believe that eventually there will be guidelines to decide what should be covered. Ideally, the services that are covered should provide a reasonable baseline for every American—one that we would be proud to tell our friends around the world about but one that is not excessive. We should cover those treatments for which there is evidence that the service is beneficial (so-called 'evidence-based benefits'). In some cases, because there will not be studies available, expert opinion (such as that currently found in many national practice guidelines) will have to be enough."[29]

However, even the list of truly beneficial services is likely to be unaffordable at some point, and then the really hard work will begin. A system such as the one tried in Oregon guided by principles such as those proposed by Emanuel will likely be developed in combination with mathematical cost effectiveness and common sense, generating a list of covered services. Payment for treatments related to diseases linked to self-defeating behavior such as smoking and overeating, as well as "futile" care at the extremes of life, will have to be balanced against paying for other effective treatments.

Who will make the decisions about which medical services are "essential"? Broad decisions regarding what will be covered cannot be reached by individuals—either by the physicians treating patients or by the patients themselves. In both cases, everyone will always want everything covered. Because it is important to take such decisions out of the realm of politics, a completely independent group—perhaps structured like the Federal Reserve—may need to be established. This group will need to test a number of principles such as those proposed above.

Once the prioritized list of services is developed, the budget will determine how far down the list is considered truly "affordable" in the system, whether this is an employer saying that this is all they will pay or funding is provided through government programs such as Medicare. How much medical care we can ultimately afford to pay for is likely to be defined by how much waste we can eliminate in the current system and how much we, as a country, decide to continue to spend on medical care.

If the services that are considered essential cannot be covered, then there are really only two choices: increase the amount each person is willing to pay into the system, or further ration the care. We must begin discussions about rationing with patients, families, professionals, and ethicists and *not* with "medical industrialists," who gain directly from prolonging life at every expense. Calling rationing the third rail doesn't help anyone. We will benefit from allowing the FDA to set high bars for value—including both cost and effectiveness—for approving new drugs and devices where low-value drugs would not be approved, allowing Medicare to consider cost in what it covers, and listening carefully to people with terminal diseases and following their wishes rather than those of their physicians.

Because this is America, those who can pay will be able to buy more care than those who cannot pay. This disparity is not unethical as long as we define an "adequate" baseline of care and provide it to everyone. Unfortunately, the definition of *adequate* depends upon where you stand. No matter what, we will eventually need to come to grips with the fact that we cannot all have it all.

## CHAPTER SUMMARY

- Medical-care rationing is happening today in the United States: the MD Anderson Cancer Center chair in the Leukemia Department estimates that 40 percent of his patients are getting less than optimal care because they can't afford the drugs they need.
- The uninsured get about half the care of the insured and have a 40 percent higher mortality rate under the age of sixty-five than the insured. This is a form of rationing.
- Oregon tried explicit rationing of Medicaid services in 1994. Doctors and patients figured out ways around it.
- The United Kingdom has the most public, widespread system for explicit rationing. The National Institute for Health and Care Excellence (NICE)

decides which drugs will be paid for by the government based on how "cost effective" they are.

- Rationing isn't done to be cruel. It's a way to allocate scarce resources. There are ethical ideas for how we can approach rationing proposed by Dr. Ezekiel Emanuel and his colleagues.
- If we decide to limit spending on ineffective care and other forms of waste, we may have enough resources to give people effective care—for the time being.
- Ultimately we will need to understand that we cannot all have it all.

## Chapter Nine

# Myth: The United States Faces a Dangerous Shortage of Doctors

There's a good chance the last time you tried to call a doctor—especially if you were trying to get an appointment with a specialist—you had to wait longer than you felt was reasonable to get an appointment. The situation probably raised a slew of questions in your mind: *How long should it take to get an appointment? Do I really need that appointment? Was my last doctor's visit really necessary? Could I be seen by a nurse instead of a doctor? Do I have a simple question that could be answered by phone or e-mail?*

Patients are aware of how difficult it is to get appointments. Many doctors agree that the situation is less than ideal, so, of course, it's become all too easy to say, *Of course we need more doctors!* But do we?

## HOW MANY DOCTORS DO WE NEED?

Interestingly, every time in the past twenty years that a surplus or shortage of doctors has been predicted, the eventual reality has looked quite different. Take, for example, predictions made during the early 1990s during the growth of the health maintenance organizations. HMOs, as they are known, were promised to improve efficiency, since they positioned primary-care physicians as gatekeepers who would need to give their patients permission to see specialists. The conventional wisdom was that HMOs would reduce unnecessary trips to specialists, so we'd wind up with a surplus of physicians. But the HMO model fell out of favor as Americans insisted on having more freedom of choice about selecting their physicians and having more direct access to specialists. The forecast excess never materialized.

Then a 2004 prediction said the United States would experience a shortage of as many of two hundred thousand physicians by 2025.[1] Where are we now? In 2017, the Association of American Medical Colleges (AAMC) projected that by 2030 any shortage would be much lower—between seven thousand and forty-three thousand primary-care physicians and between thirty-four thousand and sixty-two thousand specialists, about half of the original prediction. For the first time, the AAMC recognized that the need for specialists was much greater than previously thought, due in part to the health problems associated with an aging population.[2]

Making these kinds of forecasts is challenging work, since they need to identify from among the general population a likely pool of future physicians while accounting for the eleven or more years of education each one will have to complete after high school if they want to go into practice as a doctor. So much can change during that time frame that these sorts of projections are inaccurate at best and useless at worst. Nonetheless, let's look at where we stand now and then discuss trends we might be able to safely identify for the future.[3]

## Do We Need More Doctors Today?

How would we know whether we need more doctors? Unfortunately, some oft-quoted numbers used for predictions are not terribly helpful. Consider the ratio of physicians to the US population: We rank twenty-nine out of thirty-nine nations in the OECD, with 2.6 physicians per thousand population.[4] But it may be worth taking this measure with a grain of salt. Some of the nations with the highest numbers of physicians per capita have the worst life expectancy, like Lithuania, which ranks third in terms of number of physicians (4.3 for every one thousand residents) but 112th in life expectancy, recognizing that life expectancy has a number of other factors. We need to know more about the distribution of physicians—where they're located, how they're trained, and whether they're specialists—for this figure to be really useful.

But certain metrics do make sense. The amount of time it takes a patient to actually get an appointment with a physician is a fairly straightforward measure. In 2017, consulting firm Merritt Hawkins studied the wait times to see a physician for new patients.[5] Overall, they found a 30 percent increase in wait time from 2014 to 2017, rising from 18.5 to 24.1 days. Boston was the city with the worst delays, with wait times averaging fifty-two days, while Dallas was best, at fifteen days. The knee-jerk response among patients might be that any wait is too long. But increasingly we Americans must get used to the idea that everything cannot happen instantaneously. That being said, a referral for a possible cancer diagnosis should occur at the speed of light.

Merritt Hawkins also studies health-workforce recruiting. The years between 2012 and 2017 saw a 17 percent increase overall in physician job openings in the United States; the increase was entirely due to specialty physician positions. From these statistics, it appears that there is a physician shortage today in some specialties, in some parts of the country.[6]

## TRENDS IN PHYSICIAN SUPPLY AND DEMAND

### Supply

*The Number of Medical Students and Residents*

In 2002, based on projected physician shortages at the time, the AAMC recommended a 30 percent increase in the number of physicians graduating from medical schools—either by increasing the number of students in each class or by creating new medical schools. In 2017 that goal was reached, with 21,434 students graduating—an increase of 4,946 students over 2002 numbers—driven largely by a growing number of new US medical schools opening their doors.[7] Combined first-year enrollment at medical schools granting MD degrees and DO degrees (doctor of osteopathy—a different type of medical degree that offers the same rights and privileges as an MD) is projected to reach 30,186 students between 2020 and 2021, an increase of 55 percent compared with 2002–2003 numbers.[8] Later in this chapter, we'll discuss whether it is possible (or even desirable) to continue to increase the number of physician graduates.

After medical school, a physician must complete residency to learn hands-on how to care for patients. Hospitals, rather than medical schools, supervise and pay for residents. Residencies last from three years to six years and may then be followed by a fellowship in a subspecialty—like cardiology after studying internal medicine, for example—which lasts another two to three years. When Medicare was created in the 1960s, leaders thought there was a physician shortage, so policy makers decided Medicare would reimburse hospitals for the expense of the residents who took care of Medicare patients. In 1997, thinking there was a physician surplus, Medicare froze the number of positions it would fund. Medicare has not removed that freeze in numbers, although the payment per resident has increased. But hospitals can fund any number of residents they want. Hospitals added 8,640 first-year resident positions (a 33 percent increase) between 1997 and 2016, demonstrating that the payment by the government did not really prevent their increasing resident numbers. The arguments are beyond the scope of this discussion, but suffice it to say that some wonder whether hospitals should receive payment for residents from Medicare or other insurance companies at all.[9] Hospitals can actually see residents as cheap labor: A first-year resident works eighty hours for about $54,000,[10] and a new registered nurse makes about $64,500.[11] The resident makes $13 an hour (and can determine the care for the patient), and the nurse (who cannot) makes $31.

*Work Hours and Retirement*

For the last several years, approximately 50 percent of physicians entering practice are women. Among two-physician couples without children, men worked an average of fifty-seven hours a week, and women worked about fifty-two (10 percent fewer hours); women with toddlers aged one to two years worked 25 percent fewer hours than did women without children, and the men worked 3.5 percent fewer hours than men without children.[12] Both male and female primary-care physicians who are younger work fewer hours than their older colleagues.[13] This is not surprising: In addition to changing lifestyle preferences, our current generation of physicians must limit the time they spend in residency training to eighty hours per week. This mandate is based on evidence that medical mistakes were being made and learning suffered because of sleep deprivation—too many hours at work and not enough at home, sleeping. The new message to residents is that prolonged sleepless hours at the patient's bedside are dangerous for both the patient and the trainee. This message is a good one and will be taken forward. Meanwhile, the next generation of doctors is telling us that they want more time to have a life outside of medicine to be with their families. As a result, they're predicted to work 13 percent fewer hours than their predecessors. For all specialty categories, physician-retirement decisions are projected to have the greatest impact on supply, and more than one-third of all currently active physicians will be sixty-five or older within the next decade.[14] The take-home message on physician supply is that the total number of hours worked by physicians is likely to decrease from where we are today.

## Nurse Practitioners and Physician Assistants

By 2030, the ratio of nurse practitioners (NPs) and physician assistants (PAs) to physicians will double.[15] An analysis by the Health Resources and Services Administration projects that by that time the United States will have large surplus of primary-care NPs and PAs. This "surplus" would evaporate if NPs and PAs are able to substitute for physicians. This substitution will be entirely in the hands of state licensing boards, which by 2030 may finally realize that such substitutions mean patients receive the care they need. Virtually all studies have shown essentially no difference in the quality of care provided by nurse practitioners compared with primary-care physicians; in fact, in some studies, patient-satisfaction rates were higher for NPs.[16] It may be that the most important way to address the possible physician shortages is to permit NPs to have independent practice and be allowed to function essentially as physicians, as is currently permitted in twenty-one states.[17]

## Electronic Health Records

In the not-too-distant future, physician supply is likely to increase after time efficiencies are created with the use of electronic health records. EHRs will simplify administrative work, freeing up physicians' time so they can spend their hours reviewing and seeing complex patient cases, and with superior patient records, EHRs will keep physicians better informed with reminders of needed tests and other management so patient return visits will be more effective. In addition, time spent billing will be markedly reduced, as notes from visits and procedures entered into the EHR will be "understood" by a billing system, automatically billing patients and insurance companies. Tests and prescriptions will also be ordered automatically, based on the information in the EHR.

However, that is still mostly wishful thinking. Todays EHRs are thought to save little physician time—and in some cases doctors complain that struggling with poorly designed EHR systems takes up even *more* time. Nevertheless, there is evidence that electronic records do improve patient care. Some estimates suggest that in the next fifteen years EHRs will save time and improve physician productivity. All things being equal, this would mean a decrease in need for physicians; however, it might also mean that physicians will see the same number of patients but spend more time with each of them.[18] Time will tell.

Of course, even the best-designed EHR won't add much value without a good physician. But when it comes to trying to determine the appropriate number of physicians to treat the US population over the next twenty years, we face several inescapable realities related to demand.

## Demand for Physicians: Do We Need More?

### *Aging of the Population*

Baby boomers, born between 1946 and 1964, are graying: ten thousand of them turn sixty-five every day. According to the Population Reference Bureau, "The number of Americans aged sixty-five and older is projected to more than double from forty-six million today to more than ninety-eight million by 2060, and the sixty-five-and-older age group's share of the total population will rise to nearly 24 percent from 15 percent."[19]

### *Increased Burden of Chronic Illness*

We are living longer with chronic diseases, with 88 percent of the population over sixty-five years old having at least one chronic disease, and nearly a quarter of them experiencing at least five chronic diseases. By 2030, a third of boomers will be obese, a quarter will have diabetes, and almost half will have arthritis.[20] This increasing rate of chronic disease will also drive the need for more physicians, because it takes time to treat patients with multiple chronic diseases. Therefore, combining the number of baby boomers, the boomers' insatiable demand for immediate service, the growing number of chronic illnesses they will suffer, and our current limited ability to effectively cure chronic disease, demand for medical care is going to increase. We agree with the Association of American Medical Colleges that the number of specialists needed will exceed the number of generalists.[21]

### *Advances in Medicine*

Throughout centuries, medical science has delivered innovative therapies to improve medical care, and we can expect continued advances in medicine over the next ten years.

1. We will be better able to predict in any individual patient what diseases are likely to occur. We will then apply preventive treatment to those who are likely to benefit. The goal of better-individualized strat-

egies is to keep people alive and in the best possible health. But better health of the entire US population is not likely to be realized in the next ten years. There will be a number of preventive strategies leading to increased monitoring (for example, more tests to be sure that the prevention is "working"), and so in the near term of the next ten years or so, we are not likely to need fewer physicians on this basis.

In the longer term, prevention of an earlier disease will permit the patient to live long enough to get the next disease. It is just not known whether the next disease will require more or less physician intervention. For example, if improved medical knowledge prevents lung cancer and the patient later dies from prolonged heart failure, more physicians will be required to treat the heart condition than had the patient died quickly from the lung cancer. Of course, we want people to live longer. But prevention will likely result in the need for more physicians, not fewer, as prevention ultimately means people living longer with chronic disease. However, if dying becomes a much more acceptable and comfortable process, we may need fewer physicians as more patients and families become comfortable with the idea of hospice care.

2. Medical innovations will eventually enable us to determine in the individual patient which drugs will work best for an increasing number of diseases, such as infections and cancer. This type of personalized medicine will be effective, but it will also require more sophisticated testing, not less, leading to increased survival with chronic disease and, thus, an increased need for care.

3. In the future we will be able to truly cure more diseases. A greater understanding of the human genome will give physicians the ability to identify people who are likely to get certain diseases and then to manipulate an individual's genes to prevent the disease, either by destroying bad genes or by inserting good genes. Although this may sound like science fiction, we will actually begin to apply these sorts of advances to patient care in the next ten to twenty years. More physicians will be required to help guide this "genetic revolution." Our current doctors are not trained in the use of genetic therapy, and it is likely that this approach will be so advanced that there will be a need for new specialists in this field. The first attempts to solve single-gene problems like hemophilia or cystic fibrosis are likely to involve intensive effort with ongoing monitoring and treatment, requiring

more physicians. Eventually, the one-time fixes we'll find manipulating the patient's genes, rendering them truly disease-free, will begin to occur, hopefully allowing them to remain healthy right up until death, which will then lead to a reduced need for physicians.

4. Finally, we will have better technology—such as better imaging to show coronary heart disease and colon cancer without needing to put tubes into the patient's body—and better instruments to do basic surgery—for example, replacing heart valves by threading tubes through the arteries and veins rather than opening the chest. The shifts in these types of procedures may slightly change what, for example, heart surgeons and cardiologists do, but these changes in technology are not likely to impact the overall need for physicians until the diseases are eliminated.

## Physician-Induced and Patient-Induced Demand

Today's medical system is probably providing too many services to patients, and by some measures overtreatment accounts for 25 percent of US health care.[22] By that reasoning, when we start doing the "right things" for patients—and only doing the right things—physicians should have more time, and thus we won't need as many as we think.

For example, the need for the annual physical examination has been debated.[23] Think about it: half of primary-care visits are fifteen minutes or less. What actually happens in those visits? It is unlikely that lasting relationships are forged during that time. These well-adult checks are seen as preventive maintenance. They include work like blood-pressure checks, sometimes a cholesterol blood-level check, and, for women, a breast exam (though it's unclear whether doctors can do this better than patients). Does any of this require a physician? We speak of *physician-induced demand*, a fancy way of referring to doctors' propensity to overtreat patients. Addressing this situation could help reduce the need for physicians, but so could addressing the other side of the equation—*patient-induced demand*, such as unnecessary visits to emergency departments and physicians.

And, of course, when we have finally guaranteed health care for all Americans—or at least when we do a better job providing health care to more people—the number of physicians required will increase.

## HOW SHOULD WE APPROACH THE PHYSICIAN
## WORKFORCE NEEDS IN THE NEXT TEN YEARS?

It should be clear by now that all the unknowns make accurate prediction of physician numbers extremely difficult. Nevertheless, there are creative approaches we can take.

1. The AAMC projects a shortage of forty thousand to one hundred thousand physicians by 2030. One way to double the output of physicians would be to shorten undergraduate education and medical school to a combined four years. After graduation, armed with an MD degree, the doctor could be required to spend two years working under physician supervision in areas of the country with true physician shortages. These students would enter formal residency training at the same age they do now, with less debt and more valuable experience.[24] This proposal could reduce workforce shortages by thirty-nine thousand physicians per year if residents were sent underserved places, without churning out doctors who are too young and untrained.

2. Given that there may be a shortage of available care providers, we will have to do more than simply try to produce more physicians.

   *Task shifting* may be one answer: Originating in the United Kingdom, task shifting delegates assigned duties to those with the least training and lowest pay who can effectively perform them, freeing those "higher up the ladder" to concentrate on doing what they alone can do.[25] For example, in medicine, one can imagine task shifting from specialist to generalist to reduce demand for specialists and from general practitioners to nurse practitioners or physician assistants.

   One primary-care physician said between 80 and 85 percent of his patients "can be seen by a nurse practitioner or a physician's assistant." He continued,

   > People in their twenties and thirties face fewer health problems than kids and the elderly, except for the occasional injury or acute illness. People in their forties and fifties are also frequently lucky enough to stay generally healthy. It is only as we get into our sixties and beyond that we need an old-fashioned, close relationship with an internist again. . . . It's a wonderful thing to have a trusted relationship with a primary-care doctor. But as our society changes, we must adapt. It's

time to admit that our system isn't set up to allow a PCP for everyone.[26]

Primary-care physicians may see the writing on the wall. In one
study, 66 percent of the primary-care physicians surveyed said that
they thought students should pursue careers as nurse practitioners.
Only 56 percent recommended their own career path.[27] Primary-care
training should go in one of two directions: either expanding training
to prepare the physician to do almost anything (including emergency
medicine) in rural areas or focusing their training on coordination of
teams to care for complex patients.

An even greater "task shift" has occurred in India where technicians
are performing colonoscopies and other technicians are performing
cataract surgery with outstanding results.[28]

Another type of task shifting occurs when health-care work usually
performed by a nurse is performed by a nurse aide, as is done in the
company Garson founded, Grand-Aides USA, with an aim to "improve population health and provide appropriate access to care while
reducing unnecessary emergency, clinic, and hospital visits in adults
and children, thus reducing costs. Grand-Aides USA provides an innovative health-care-delivery program with caring, experienced nurse
extenders making home visits to develop a trusting relationship, con-
necting the patient and care team quickly and cost-effectively."[29]

Grand-Aides are usually certified nurse aides and can be community
health workers. Under close supervision by a nurse, Grand-Aides use
home visits with portable telemedicine to provide transitional (hospital discharge) and chronic-disease management. In patients with heart
failure (and the usual comorbidities including diabetes, chronic ob-
structive pulmonary disease, and renal disease) care with Grand-Aides
has shown an 82 percent reduction in all-cause thirty-day readmissions (to 2.8 percent), a 91 percent reduction in thirty-day all-cause
emergency-department visits, and similar highly significant reductions
in unnecessary admissions, readmissions, and ED visits at six months.
Medication adherence was 92 percent. Length of stay decreased from
9.0 to 6.2 days.[30]

The final type of task-shift is to patients themselves, to have them
caring for themselves so that, ideally, they don't need a physician, thus
reducing demand for physicians. An estimated 40 percent of life ex-

pectancy is determined by behavior, including overeating, smoking, drinking excessive amounts of alcohol, drug abuse, violence, and automobile fatalities.[31] Additionally, patients can limit their visits to physicians and EDs for minor illnesses. Finally, they can both improve their medication adherence (ultimately requiring less care) and reduce the requests for unnecessary drugs.

3.  Though we think there's mixed evidence of a physician shortage in the future, one thing we know for sure is that right now we have a shortage of practitioners in rural areas that must be addressed. We know that physicians raised in rural areas are willing to practice in rural areas, as are those who have been given hefty financial incentives to do so.[32] The shortage can be addressed somewhat by permitting independent practice of nurse practitioners—in other words, allowing them to practice like doctors. They are a key part of the solution, because we know NPs are more likely to work in rural areas than physicians.[33]

    We also know there are shortages of providers in inner cities. People who are disabled and live in low-income areas of cities may be a mere few miles away from a physician as the crow flies but may have tremendous difficulty getting to a physician's office. Any initiatives aimed at rural access to care must also address the needs found in inner cities.[34] Technology can help. Telemedicine directly into the homes of patients will certainly improve access to care.

4.  The Affordable Care Act did little to improve access to health care. *Access* is defined as the right person in the right place at the right time. Lawmakers should create a commission to understand the changing needs in medicine and coordinate with workforce commissions in each state to better understand local supply and demand. A national commission can also serve as a clearinghouse of the best ideas across the country for addressing practitioner shortages.

    These commissions can be the eyes and ears of the country's patients, honing predictions of supply and demand yearly and empowered to fund incentives for practitioners to go into needed specialties. They can provide funding for professional schools and residencies that would stimulate greater numbers of physicians and nurses being trained in specialties that are needed. They could also play a role in expanding the National Health Service Corps, which serves underserved areas by offering practitioners larger financial incentives to practice in underserved areas for longer periods of time.

## THE BOTTOM LINE

There is currently a physician shortage, especially in rural areas and inner cities. This shortage may not turn out to be as serious as some suggest, and it can be reduced through several innovative approaches, such as relying more on nurse practitioners and rethinking the way we train and place doctors. Given the unknowns regarding future demand for medical services, federal and state workforce commissions should continuously update projections and be given the ability to provide financial incentives for physicians—and medical students—to enter a needed specialty in underserved areas.

## CHAPTER SUMMARY

- The United States is currently experiencing a shortage of doctors, especially in rural areas, though the shortage isn't as dramatic as it once was predicted to be.
- The Association of American Medical Colleges currently predicts a shortage of forty thousand to one hundred thousand physicians by 2030. The need for specialists is, and will be, greater than the need for primary-care physicians. US medical schools can't educate enough doctors quickly enough.
- We can address much of the projected shortage through *task shifting*, where generalists do the work currently done by some specialists and nurse practitioners perform much of the work of primary-care doctors. The final task shift is for patients to assume greater responsibility for their own wellness.
- Telemedicine for rural and even some urban areas will be an important addition to the mix of solutions to address the coming shortage.
- Improved projections of workforce need as well as creation of appropriate incentives can also help address the workforce challenges and ward off a dangerous shortage.

# Chapter Ten

# Myth: The Current Malpractice System Protects Patients

The current medical malpractice system is intended to help patients, identify doctors who are making dangerous mistakes, and ultimately improve the quality of medical care. But the sad reality is that the malpractice system largely fails at each of these goals. There has to be a better way.

Before discussing solutions, let's make clear what we mean by *malpractice*. For malpractice to have occurred, first, there needs to be negligence. Specifically, that means a physician failed to provide treatment that is in line with the *medical standard of care*—usually defined as care that a "reasonably competent physician, with a similar background and in the same medical community, would have provided under similar circumstances."[1] Second, for there to be negligence, a patient needs to have been injured.

As we think about ways to improve the health-care system, one question we have to ask is whether this part of the system relating to malpractice—which is intended to help patients—really does that. The goal of malpractice is to help patients recover financially if they've been harmed by a negligent physician. Specifically, the financial recovery of a medical malpractice lawsuit is intended to provide for

1. economic damages from loss of work, to pay the patient for estimated income they would have received had the injury not occurred,
2. economic damages needed to pay for medical care expenses, and
3. noneconomic damages for things such as pain and suffering.

The idea surely seems reasonable, and occasionally patients who are truly victims of negligence are appropriately paid. As we will see, there are short-comings in the system. For example, we might wonder, *Are those who file malpractice suits actual victims of negligence? And are people who are actual victims for negligence claiming malpractice? When they are victims of negligence, are they appropriately compensated? Are doctors who commit repeated acts of negligence educated to prevent mistakes in the future? Do they lose their licenses if they don't improve?*

The current malpractice system does not guarantee a yes to any of these questions.

## DOES THE SYSTEM HELP INJURED PATIENTS?

Only about 8 percent of malpractice cases go to trial, and of those cases the patient wins only about 25 percent of the time. Why are these numbers so low?[2] Let's consider two possibilities.

1. It's possible that the judgments are correct and that the overwhelming majority of the time there was no true medical malpractice. But it's difficult to know whether this is true. Even if we get experts to look back on malpractice suits, we know that they don't agree.
2. The process itself is broken, and we see examples of its failing *both* patients and doctors. On the patient side, plaintiff's attorneys know that malpractice cases are challenging to win. As a result, they tend to pick cases that are most likely to bring large awards. In the majority of cases, the plaintiff lawyers are only paid if they win. Therefore, law-yers take one-third to even two-thirds of the plaintiff's winnings. Cer-tainly some portion of the payment is needed to cover the expenses of other cases that they are going to lose and for which they get no payment. In our system, this means that the low-income person with no health insurance who has a valid claim and simply wants to have their $10,000 medical bills paid may not be able to find an attorney willing to take their case. The economics of making that patient whole don't work out for the patient.

Twenty-six states have laws that limit or cap damage claims. Some states limit noneconomic damages (so called "pain and suffering"), while others limit the entire award.[3] "The rate of paid medical-malpractice claims has declined significantly, dropping nearly 56 percent between 1992 and 2014 with the caps on awards being among the most likely causes."[4] This makes it even more challenging for patients to find attorneys willing to take their case, resulting in fewer claims filed.

The system fails physicians, too, since it relies on those who don't know much about medicine—juries—to weigh in on enormously complicated health issues. For example, in one case known personally to Garson, a physician was found guilty of malpractice, but this verdict was unexpected, as it turns out, by both sides. In questioning the jury foreman after the award, the doctor's attorney was told that the jury "trusted the plaintiff's attorney because the attorney was born with one arm and must have worked very hard to overcome his handicap" and "the defendant doctor"—who had been absent for three days of the ten-day trial to care for his patients—"must not have cared about this patient or he would have been here every day." Enough said.

## CAN THE SYSTEM IDENTIFY NEGLIGENCE?

Only about 20 percent of actual negligence committed by health-care providers gets recorded.[5] That means we have physicians practicing today who have been negligent and not identified. Their patients likely have no idea who these physicians are. However, we know that only 15–20 percent of malpractice claims appear to involve actual negligence.[6]

Congress created the National Practitioner Data Bank for public access to examine any physician's record of lawsuits.[7] One in every three physicians has been sued.[8] Therefore, it seems clear that a physician's being sued is not necessarily an indicator of their poor quality medical care. Nonetheless, a repeat offender does seem to predict more lawsuits. "Just 1 percent of doctors were linked to 32 percent of malpractice settlements paid." The more claims a doctor settled, the higher the likelihood they would pay in the future. "The highest-risk doctors—those with six or more paid settlement claims—have more than twelve times the risk of a recurring settlement payment."[9]

With our present system, nobody wins. When a physician is sued, it is devastating, generally leading to self-doubt that may persist for years. In the cases where some self-examination is healthy—when the physician actually was negligent—this is perhaps a good thing. But for doctors who have acted appropriately, tried their best, and done nothing wrong despite a bad medical outcome, the malpractice process can be sufficiently traumatic that they decide leave the profession. That's not good for doctors or patients.

## HOW ARE DAMAGES CALCULATED?

When patients do win their lawsuits, the math that goes into determining the amount they are paid can be complicated. Most often damages are based on the prediction that the patient would have continued to work into the future. In fact, the plaintiff—the patient—may collect the damages and continue to work. The plaintiff can also seek disability benefits from the government, regardless of whether the patient has a private insurer who pays the bills— although not all states allow this type of double payment. So what's the problem with all of this?

For starters, when there is an award that has been carefully justified and calculated, the patient often goes home with less than half of the actual amount. In many cases, most of the damages are paid out as attorney expenses (which we touched on above). If we're really meticulously doing the math to ensure that patients are made whole, then those fees seem laughably inadequate. For example, if the patient is fifty-five years old and earning a salary of $75,000, we might expect the following damages:

- $750,000 for missing a decade of work until retirement at sixty-five,
- medical care expenses of $100,000 ($10,000 per year until Medicare begins paying when the patient turns sixty-five), and
- noneconomic damages of $150,000 for pain and suffering.

There are added calculations that go into the time period over which the money is paid, but for our example this comes out to a grand total of $1,000,000. If the attorney takes $600,000, how is the person who cannot work going to pay rent and other expenses? In this example, it would seem that the attorney's $600,000 fee should be above and beyond the actual amount awarded to the patient. Attorneys should certainly be compensated at whatever level seems fair, but it would be more reasonable to make this payment known up front, rather than deducting payment from an award that has been rigorously calculated to address the actual needs of the patient. Having lawyers' fees as an add-on to the damages rather than as a deduction from the damages is already done in other types of lawsuits, such as civil-rights cases, and it should be done as well in medical malpractice.

## DOES THE SYSTEM IMPROVE QUALITY OF CARE?

Earlier in this book, we discussed the elements that account for quality health care. Let's consider whether our current system for handling medical malpractice actually improves quality of care.

### Safety

By one estimate, 27 percent of *adverse events*—things that go wrong—in a hospital are due to negligence.[10] Complications or even death may occur in many procedures. For example, surgical procedures generally carry a 3–4 percent risk of infection.[11] "Sterile techniques, cleaning the area, and antibiotics may be used in an attempt to guard against infection. Despite such care, infection can occur. This would be an adverse event but not one necessarily due to a medical error. It would instead be a risk inherent in the practice of medicine."[12]

In one study of more than twenty-seven thousand events in a hospital thought to be due to negligence, only 2 percent resulted in malpractice claims.[13] In other words, a large number of medical errors and avoidable injuries are never addressed within the malpractice system. In many of these cases, a malpractice suit may have given the physician a chance to learn from their mistake or to be accountable to their peers. But 98 percent of the time, that didn't happen. Meanwhile, it is not likely that safety will improve even if the number of malpractice claims were to double from 2 percent to 4 percent; the overwhelming majority of the cases would still go unaddressed. It seems that the legal system is not going to be a good way to improve medical safety overall.

### Effectiveness

Physicians in specialties that handle higher-risk procedures, like obstetricians and neurosurgeons, are either leaving the practice of medicine or moving to states with more favorable caps on "noneconomic" damages—meaning that they're choosing to practice in places where there is a limit to what can be paid for pain and suffering. This reduction in specialists in states with unfavorable malpractice laws creates real access problems for those needing care and is a problem in rural regions, where some patients may have to drive 150 miles to see an obstetrician and deliver their baby.

## Efficiency

The United States spends $10 billion per year on the direct cost of malpractice litigation—including about $3.2 billion for actual health-care reimbursement (economic damages) and about $2.6 billion on pain and suffering. About $2 billion pays for plaintiff lawyer expense, about $1 billion for defense lawyer expense and then another $1.2 billion on overhead.[14] These are huge costs that add up, and they contribute to our nation's ballooning problem with overspending on health care.

## Defensive Medicine

The expenses associated with *defensive medicine*—or when doctors conduct unnecessary tests and procedures out of fear of a malpractice lawsuit—also increase the cost of medical care in the country. Part of the difficulty in coming up with a number for what defensive medicine costs is that it's not so simple to determine when, exactly, a doctor is performing defensive medicine. One study has concluded that it was not possible to tell from reading any chart (medical record) whether a physician ordered a test out of fear of malpractice.[15]

So why not just ask physicians whether they're practicing defensive medicine? In one study, physicians were asked about the extent to which fear of malpractice figured into their medical decisions. They answered that there are a number of reasons that they order tests and procedures: it turned out that about 13 percent of the cost of tests and hospital admissions were associated, at least partly, with a fear of getting sued—or defensive medicine. But just 2.9 percent of costs were ordered *completely* because of defensive medicine. In another study, sample cases were provided to physicians who were asked what caused them to order certain tests or procedures. Malpractice was third on the list, behind "to obtain clinical information" and "to do what others in the community do" not out of fear of malpractice but just because "everyone does it." Fourth, after "malpractice," was "patient expectations." The authors examining the study pointed out that this list did not ask physicians how often they order tests and procedures "to make money."[16] Yet, in another study, 71 percent of physicians believed that "other physicians" (not referring to themselves) "were more likely to perform unnecessary procedures when they profited from them."[17]

What do we take from this discussion of defensive medicine? It is difficult to assess the cost of defensive medicine. Unfortunately, the only way to find out whether someone is practicing defensive medicine is to ask, but it seems that, at most, about 5–8 percent of medical decisions are made primarily due to malpractice concerns.[18] Therefore, the extent to which defensive medicine drives up national medical costs may be overstated. And so, when asked why physicians do certain tests and procedures, blaming fear of malpractice is an easier explanation than considering the study that found "71 percent of physicians were more likely to perform unnecessary procedures when they profited from them."[19]

## TRYING TO FIX A BROKEN SYSTEM

The malpractice system doesn't work on multiple fronts. Why? Partly because each part of a charge of malpractice involves people who try to be objective but may not always be:

- The patient has been injured and is angry.
- The doctor is hurt, defensive, and angry.
- The lawyers have a job to do.
- The jury may not understand the fine points of medicine.
- Expert witnesses each have their own biases, based on their background and, unfortunately, who is paying them.[20]

How do we overcome all of this? Here we offer a three-point solution.

First, we need a system to call out obvious malpractice before it goes to court. Physicians must be encouraged to admit their mistakes and apologize to the patient and family. This surely does not always happen. For example, a recent study that found that 77 percent of three hundred primary-care doctors admitted they would not fully disclose to a patient when there had been a delayed breast cancer diagnosis.[21] Fortunately, a new approach is being promoted by the federal Agency for Healthcare Research and Quality. CANDOR—or Communication and Optimal Resolution[22]—aims to get hospitals to proactively apologize to the victims of serious medical errors and offer fair payment for their injuries. According to a study at the University of Michigan, full disclosure of medical errors resulted in its hospital system reducing the number of lawsuits it faced by half and saving the hospital system $2 million in lawsuits. This supports the principle that doing the right thing and admitting the error is often the best approach.

The most glaring examples of malpractice—amputating the wrong leg, for example—can be settled quickly. In less obvious cases, we can compare what happened with the national practice guidelines physicians are supposed to adhere to. A physician who does something that is not indicated in a guideline resulting in patient injury could be considered to have acted negligently—as long as the guideline actually applied to that patient. In such a clear case of negligence, the physician would need to apologize for the injury, and the patient would receive payment according to a determined schedule of damages related to seriousness of the injury, the likelihood of disability, and some amount for their pain and suffering. The need for attorneys in these cases would be reduced. Much of the time patients or families reach out to an attorney simply to get answers about why a loved one has been injured or died when the hospital and risk managers refuse to tell them. [23]

The second way we can turn around our malfunctioning medical-malpractice system is through creating specialty *health courts*, in which a judge or tribunal with knowledge of medicine and experience in malpractice decides the case rather than a jury. [24] Experienced health-care judges would work full time in these types of medical-malpractice courts, and two or three nonbiased experts paid by the court would testify to ensure that all sides of the case are represented and to guard against any conflicts of interest. The fact of the matter is that the judicial system is not the best place for the truth of malpractice cases to emerge, and we need a system in which *both* doctors and patients can be confident that fair, correct decisions will be made.

Moreover, the majority of states have implemented caps on remuneration for pain and suffering, often at about $250,000. [25] Other limits have taken hold as well, such as maximum damages, including the recovery for direct medical-care costs and loss of work. Interestingly, it appears that the amount of overall awards in lawsuits in these states may not actually decrease, since the cap on damages becomes the new standard for what is demanded even though the patient might have asked for less. We need a system in which patients are awarded what they are entitled to receive rather than what legislators think makes sense.

The third way we can reform our medical-malpractice system is removing the decision of a physician's competence to practice from the legal system. Physicians should review the performance of other physicians long before a lawsuit is threatened. As we discuss elsewhere in this book, more outcome data are becoming available regarding physicians' quality performance, so, fortunately, physicians increasingly have the opportunity to evaluate for themselves how their peers are doing, using national guidelines and standards. It may be a few more years until data are accurate enough for us to make determinations at the level of the individual physician—as opposed to groups of physicians—but when the data are available, those physicians with borderline outcomes should be identified by colleagues, hospitals, health-insurance plans, state boards of medicine, or all four. Programs must be put in place that help those clinicians who are deficient. And in those cases where the medical care remains of unacceptable quality, physicians must not permit their fellow physician to practice.

## CHAPTER SUMMARY

- Only about 8 percent of malpractice cases go to trial, and of those cases, the patient wins about 25 percent of the time. The math? Patients win 2 percent of malpractice cases.
- The system doesn't match negligence and malpractice. Only about 20 percent of actual negligence committed by health-care providers gets recorded. However, only 15–20 percent of malpractice claims appear to involve actual negligence.
- One in every three physicians is sued. Therefore, getting sued is not a very good indicator of a physician's quality. A repeat offender does seem to predict more lawsuits, however, with 32 percent of medical malpractice payouts linked to a mere 1 percent of doctors.
- About 5–8 percent of medical decisions are made by physicians primarily due to fear of malpractice—so-called *defensive medicine*. It is difficult to assess when defensive medicine is being practiced, since the medical record does not shed light on this question; the only way is to directly ask a physician why they did or did not do something, and there are usually multiple reasons for any one medical decisions. Physicians say that that 71 percent of their colleagues are more likely to perform unnecessary procedures when they profit from them.
- What to do? The law is not the right way to deal with doctors who need improvement. Nonetheless, where a physician has been found to be negligent and convicted of malpractice, after they have been instructed on improvement, if the medical care they provide remains of unacceptable quality as judged by their peers, the physician must not be permitted to practice.

## Chapter Eleven

# Myth: In the United States There Is a Safety Net of Government Health Programs for the Poor

In the first chapter of this book, we told the story of Ginny, Garson's young patient with a heart-rhythm problem. Ginny lived well for years, thanks to medical care she received through Medicaid, the government health-insurance program that covers children in low-income families.

Unfortunately, the worst thing that ever happened to Ginny was turning nineteen years old. Why? That's the age we, as a society, have decided people no longer need affordable health care, and we leave young people to fend for themselves. When Ginny turned nineteen, she aged out of Medicaid in Texas and was no longer eligible. She didn't have a job that provided health insurance. And she didn't have enough money to pay her health-care costs out of pocket.

She died because she couldn't afford the medication that kept her heart beating at a normal rate. She was one of the "forgottens" when Medicaid was created. Of course, they thought, people over nineteen would normally have health insurance through their job. And she surely wasn't a "forgotten" by her parent, friends, and doctors.

In this chapter, we'll explain how health care is provided—and, in many cases, *isn't* provided—by the public system. We deal with the "private" or "commercial" insurance system in the next chapter. Here we explain how public insurance worked before 2013, in the days before the Affordable Care Act ("Obamacare"). The law was passed in 2010, but given the rollout of the various phases of the ACA, the changes did not really begin until 2013.[1] Then we will discuss what happened to US health care after the law, which aimed to expand the safety net, took effect. Importantly, we'll explain why the ACA wasn't more successful.

## DOES HEALTH INSURANCE MATTER?

The stark fact is that uninsured people between ages nineteen and sixty-four have 40 percent higher mortality than those with health insurance.[2] This isn't a coincidence; it's due in large part to the fact that these people are often blocked from accessing the US health-care system due to their inability to pay.

We know that "25 percent of adults without insurance go without health care, compared to just 4 percent of those with coverage. Uninsured adults who are younger than sixty-five (and thus ineligible for Medicare) are less likely than their insured peers to get preventive care, such as blood pressure checks and cancer screenings. And when the uninsured *do* get that preventative care, they're less likely to get the needed follow-up."[3] For example, uninsured women with breast cancer were 2.6 times more likely to be diagnosed at a later stage and 60 percent more likely to die from the disease than women with health insurance.[4] "Uninsured people with diabetes are six times more likely to skip needed health care because of cost compared with those who were continuously insured."[5] The uninsured are three times more likely to postpone needed care for pregnancy. Examples like these are common. Clearly the uninsured don't get the care they need. Providing a safety net for them is lifesaving.[6]

## WHO WERE THE UNINSURED IN 2013?

Back before Obamacare went into effect, no matter how poor you were, if you were between the ages of nineteen and sixty-four, for all practical purposes, there was no guaranteed health care in the United States. At that time, 49 percent of people in the United States obtained health insurance from their or a family member's employer; 32 percent received health insurance through public programs such as Medicare, and 4 percent bought their own insurance, leaving 15 percent uninsured.[7] Forty-four million Americans were uninsured, which, to put it in perspective, exceeds the population of Canada and is larger than the combined population of twenty-four states.[8] This huge number matters because of just how important health insurance is to being healthy. For many people, like Ginny, going without health insurance can be a literal death sentence.

But who exactly were these people? What were their circumstances? You may be surprised to know that the overwhelming majority of them—75 percent—had at least one full-time worker in their family. Another 11 percent had a part-time worker. These people were not lazy. They were not trying to game the system. In fact, there's a pretty easy explanation for why many of these people lacked insurance: 74 percent of them worked for an employer that didn't offer it.[9]

Ethnic minorities were the most likely to be uninsured. About 17 percent of Hispanic people were uninsured, along with 12 percent of African Americans, compared to 8 percent of Caucasians. And the uninsured were younger, with 16 percent of twenty-six- to thirty-four-year-olds lacking insurance. This likely wasn't by choice. There was a popular belief about these so-called "invincibles," who supposedly went without insurance because they believed their youth made them indestructible and didn't need insurance.[10] In fact, they went without it because they worked for businesses that did not offer health insurance and they could not afford it on their own.[11] This finding is backed up by the data from the yearly consumer survey conducted by the Texas Medical Center's Health Policy Institute, which finds that almost as many people between the ages of eighteen and thirty-four (82 percent) consider health insurance very important as those between forty-five and sixty-four (87 percent).[12]

## HOW WAS HEALTH CARE COVERED PRIOR TO 2013, WHEN THE AFFORDABLE CARE ACT TOOK HOLD?

In order to understand why we had so many uninsured people in the United States at that time, we first need to understand how health-care coverage was provided in the United States in 2013 prior to the ACA. For now, we will discuss the role of public health insurance in providing access and coverage to health services (we will discuss employer-based insurance in chapter 12). In 2013, as now, there were four major government programs that provide health coverage:

1. Medicare was created in 1965 and covered almost everyone over the age of sixty-five—approximately forty-one million people in 2013.[13]

Medicare underwent no changes with the ACA. Medicare covers people in some very specific categories, including those who are blind, have chronic kidney disease, or are permanently disabled. Medicare is paid to the federal government primarily through taxes on employers and employees. Patients on Medicare must pay a deductible (the total amount of their health-care costs payable before Medicare starts to pay) and coinsurance (the percent of the bill that the patient pays). It offers coverage of outpatient prescription drugs in relation to patient income. Average out-of-pocket spending with co-pays and deductibles for a Medicare beneficiary is $5,503 per year. If Social Security is all a person has to live on, this amount of Medicare spending eats up an average of 41 percent of their income.[14] Many patients have additional insurance called Medigap, which pays for co-pays and deductibles as well as services like vision, dental, hearing, and other types of health care not covered by Medicare.

2. Medicaid, which covered approximately fifty-five million people in 2013, was created in 1965 to provide health-care coverage for those with low incomes. The basic part of Medicaid has not changed with the ACA. Medicaid is a shared program between federal and state governments and receives funds from both. Depending upon the average income of people in the state, the federal government pays 50–76 percent of the total costs of the Medicaid program, with states picking up the rest.

   Basic Medicaid mostly covers people at each end of the age spectrum: those below nineteen and over sixty-five. Children are about 49 percent of the program's recipients. Importantly, Medicaid does not provide a safety net for adults between the ages of nineteen and sixty-four. In this age group, only mothers of Medicaid-eligible children making so little money as to be essentially unemployed are covered. Childless adults are not covered, no matter how poor they are.

   In addition to poor children, basic Medicaid covers several other categories of people: low-income pregnant women (27 percent of recipients), disabled adults under age sixty-five (15 percent of recipients), and some elderly and poor, known as *dual eligibles* (covered "dually" by Medicare and Medicaid) (9 percent of recipients).

   The decision of how poor one needs to be to receive basic Medicaid coverage is made by the federal government and is related to the federal poverty level—or the FPL—the way the United States measures poverty.

The poverty level varies by size of the family. For example, back in 2013 a single person earning $11,490 or less in a year was said to fall below the FPL; for a family of four, the FPL was $23,550.[15] By those metrics, 45.3 million people were living in poverty in the United States in 2013.[16] Basic Medicaid coverage is based on a person's income relative to the poverty level. For a family of four with a child between the ages of six to eighteen, the child would be eligible for Medicaid if the family made less than 100 percent of poverty—or less than $23,550.

3. The Children's Health Insurance Program—or CHIP—was created by Congress in 1997 to provide federal matching funds to help states expand health-care coverage to the nation's uninsured children. In 2013 as now, CHIP covered six million children,[17] filling in gaps in coverage for those younger than nineteen years old whose parents earn "too much" money to be eligible for Medicaid but still fall below 200 percent of the poverty level. In other words, drawing on one of our examples above, a family of four making $47,100 per year—or twice the income that would put them below the FPL—would not be eligible for Medicaid but would likely still struggle to make ends meet and need the extra assistance CHIP provides.[18] CHIP also covers about 370,000 pregnant women annually.[19] Like basic Medicaid, CHIP is paid for by the states and federal government, but the federal government's funding match was greater in CHIP than in Medicaid. In most situations, when state budgets expand, basic Medicaid and CHIP programs also expand their budgets, and alternately, when state budgets tighten, basic Medicaid and CHIP services are reduced, leaving previously covered individuals without health insurance. This is exactly the wrong way to fund basic Medicaid and CHIP, since in tough times people need more Medicaid, not less.

4. The Department of Veterans Affairs program in 2013 covered almost nine million people, including those retired from military service and their dependents. It is the largest health-care system in the United States, providing all types of care throughout 150 medical centers (with at least one in each state), 820 VA Community-Based Outpatient Clinics, and three VA Vet Centers, providing counseling, suicide prevention, and other services.[20]

5. Public hospitals, owned and operated by states, counties, or cities, account for about 20 percent (983) of all hospitals in the United States.[21] They comprise a crucial part of the safety net—for both hospital and outpatient care—for the uninsured and underinsured and frequently are sites of training for medical students and residents. About 40 percent of trauma care and 63 percent of burns in urban areas are handled by these hospitals.[22]

6. The "safety net of safety nets" are the federally qualified health centers (FQHC), sometimes called community clinics.[23] These are outpatient clinics placed in areas of need defined by either a lack of providers or high numbers of uninsured. They generally care for anyone under 200 percent of the poverty level and also see patients covered by Medicaid, Medicare, or commercial insurance. They charge patients based on ability to pay. In addition to emergency departments, FQHCs are where the uninsured largely receive health care. In 2013, the ten thousand FQHCs saw more than 24.3 million patients with a budget slightly higher than $5 billion.[24] While they did dispense certain prescription drugs, most FQHCs do not have access to specialists or ability to pay for hospitalization; some are not within travel distance of a public hospital. Therefore, those with chronic diseases have a problem if their condition extends beyond the scope the primary-care physicians working at the FQHC can provide.

## WITH ALL OF THESE PUBLIC PROGRAMS, HOW COME THERE ARE SO MANY UNINSURED PEOPLE?

In 2013 as now, with basic Medicaid, the majority of uninsured in the United States are between the ages of nineteen and sixty-four and are not eligible for basic Medicaid—no matter how poor.[25] Additionally, some of the uninsured are eligible for coverage but for various reasons do not apply. In 2013, 3.7 million people eligible for basic Medicaid still remained uninsured.[26] Why? Some states have complex and lengthy applications for Medicaid that must be completed in person with proof of in-state residency. In addition, proof of age, income, and assets with all the various documents like birth certificates, passports, tax forms, and wage slips must be provided; applicants often are turned away if any of the information is missing. In some states, this procedure had to be repeated every six months.

As well, Medicaid reimburses physicians only about 70 percent of the amount that Medicare will pay.[27] Across the United States, about a third of physicians refuse to see Medicaid patients because of the low reimbursement.[28] Physicians have sued the federal government to prevent any further reduction in Medicaid payment. However, on March 31, 2015, the US Supreme Court decided, in *Armstrong v. Exceptional Child Center, Inc.*, that Medicaid providers do not have the right to sue Medicaid agencies regarding payment rates.[29]

## WHAT HAS HAPPENED TO THE SAFETY NET SINCE 2013?

In 2013, forty-four million people in the United States were uninsured.[30] The Affordable Care Act worked to reduce that number by allowing people with incomes of up to 400 percent of FPL to be eligible for "expanded" Medicaid or have greater access to commercial insurance plans. What did *not* change a great deal was the care and coverage provided by Medicare, CHIP, the VA, public hospitals, and FQHCs—although they did get increased funding—which means many of the pre-2013 problems we discussed above remain problems today.

Due to improved funding for the uninsured (which we'll discuss below), especially in the states that expanded Medicaid, the pressure on public hospitals and FQHCs decreased somewhat, but they still face challenges: since they were so overcrowded pre-ACA, they are now "merely" crowded. The ACA included these specific reforms:

1. In the ACA as originally passed, Congress expanded Medicaid to cover all people in every state, including childless adults, who earn less than 138 percent of the poverty level. This was a huge expansion in coverage for uninsured Americans and a win for those who advocate for them. In 2013, 21.3 million were slated for Medicaid coverage (by 2022).[31]

   The original ACA had a provision that said if states did not expand Medicaid to the entire newly eligible population, they would lose *all* their Medicaid funding. In June 2012, the US Supreme Court, in *National Federation of Independent Business v. Sebelius*, ruled that threatening to take away all Medicaid funding—including basic Medicaid—was too coercive and so struck down this provision, making Medicaid expansion optional.[32]

Critics of that ruling say it's one of the main reasons the ACA has not been as effective as would have been hoped. As of 2018, thirty-two states and the District of Columbia had expanded Medicaid, with a total of 16.3 million new enrollees. Of these, about 75 percent are low-income adults, who now make up 15 percent of all those covered by Medicaid. Importantly, about a quarter of new enrollees were previously eligible but only signed up for Medicaid in the wake of expansion—likely in part due to increased awareness of their or their children's coverage. Overall, Medicaid expansion added about 30 percent to Medicaid roles throughout the country.[33]

Lawmakers in states opting out of Medicaid expansion have argued it would be too costly. For example, in Texas, to cover the additional two million people who would be covered by a Medicaid expansion, the state would have to pay 10 percent of the cost—or $3.3 billion per year—and the federal government, 90 percent—or $29.5 billion.[34] With a Medicaid expansion, Texas would end up paying $1,650 per new enrollee—about 33 percent of the average $5,048 per person it pays now for children, pregnant women, the disabled, and dual eligibles (who receive both Medicare and Medicaid coverage). While this might sound like a great deal, states still need to find that extra money.[35] Additionally, some states just don't want to provide more money to this group of people. One of the most common arguments against Medicaid expansion is that these uninsured people should simply work and earn enough to pay for their own insurance. But, as we have already seen, the vast majority of people in the United States who are not covered by insurance are already working.

2. The second change the ACA made was to subsidize insurance costs for people earning less than 400 percent of the poverty level so they could buy health insurance in state *marketplace exchanges*—with the goal of eventually having twenty-five million people purchasing insurance in the exchanges by 2020.[36]

Of course, the premiums represent only part of the cost for the insured. The deductible is what *really* made buying insurance in the marketplace unaffordable for so many, despite the subsidies. One of the reasons the ACA hasn't been as effective as many might have hoped is because it offers no deductible assistance for those earning more than 250 percent of FPL for a single person—not a whole lot to exist on *and* pay for health care.

If an individual's or family's income is *less* than 250 percent of FPL, the amount of money they must spend out of pocket before their insurance will kick in and begin paying for their medical bills is capped at a maximum—that is, they would not have to pay beyond a certain dollar amount per year. A single person at 250 percent FPL makes $28,725 per year, putting that person's spending cap at 8.6 percent of income.[37] We will see in the next chapter that people earning incomes don't find that level of spending to be affordable at all.

In 2017 the uninsured rate in the United States was 11.7 percent— about thirty million people—and rising, as premiums and deductibles increase. While that's fewer people without insurance than pre-ACA, it's still too many. These people were uninsured not because they didn't want the insurance but because they couldn't afford it.

In 1977, in one of his final speeches, former vice president Hubert Humphrey described the challenge we face today: "The moral test of government is how that government treats those who are in the dawn of life, the children; those who are in the twilight of life, the elderly; and those in the shadows of life, the sick, the needy, and the handicapped."[38]

By this measure, our society has not done well.

## CHAPTER SUMMARY

- We should care whether people have insurance because the uninsured have 40 percent higher mortality than the insured.
- If you think this issue doesn't affect you, think again. What would you do if you lose your job—and your employment-based coverage—and had to pay for health care out of pocket?

  - Depending on where you live, if you aren't wealthy and lose your job, you might be unable to get health care.

- A job doesn't guarantee health care, as about half of small businesses don't offer health insurance. Three-quarters of the uninsured had at least one full-time worker in their family. So, getting a job might not help get insurance coverage.
- Before the Affordable Care Act was passed, even the poorest of the poor in the United States had no assistance in getting health-care coverage if

they were a childless adult between ages nineteen and sixty-four—which meant forty-four million were uninsured. Despite what some people believe, Medicaid did not cover these people.

- As part of Obamacare, childless adults earning less than 138 percent of the federal poverty level—or $16,086 for a single person—were slated to get Medicaid coverage. But the Supreme Court made this coverage optional for states to provide. And so as of 2018, thirty-two states and Washington, D.C., have expanded Medicaid to cover this population. The rest didn't.
- Those who make 100–400 percent ($11,600–$46,600 for a single person) of FPL are eligible for some insurance subsidies. But with deductibles more than $6,000 in many cases, many still could not afford to buy the insurance.
- In 2017, the uninsured rate was 11.7 percent—about thirty million uninsured and rising, as premiums and deductibles increase.[39] While that's less than the pre-ACA total, it's still too many people who are uninsured—and not because they don't want insurance but because they can't afford it.
- No, there is *not* a safety net of US government health programs for the poor.

*Chapter Twelve*

# Myth: People Who Work Can Afford Health Insurance

During a television interview, White House advisor Kellyanne Conway offered her policy prescription for how the country could solve the unmet needs of those who lack health insurance. Those people, she explained, should just work—problem solved. "If they are able-bodied and they want to work, then they'll have employer-sponsored benefits like you and I do," she said.[1]

## MOST OF THE UNINSURED WORK

It seems that Conway, like many Americans, believes all employers provide their workers with health insurance. But, in fact, fewer than half of private-sector establishments in the United States offer health insurance to their employees.[2] About 85 percent of the uninsured come from working families, with 75 percent holding a full-time job.[3] How can that be? Seventy-four percent of nonelderly uninsured workers are employed by businesses that don't offer health insurance.[4] It's a common misconception that those on Medicaid don't work. Actually, most of them do. But their employers don't provide them with insurance, and purchasing insurance on their own is so expensive that it may be unaffordable, especially for those with low incomes. Unless policy makers face this fact, it will be impossible to fix health care in this country.

The working uninsured are people you encounter every day who know your name. They work at your dry cleaners, your favorite restaurants, the gas station you visit on the way home from work, and even some department stores where you go shopping.

In this chapter, we deal with private or "commercial" insurance, whether provided by an employer or purchased by an individual. We first consider the time before the provisions of Affordable Care Act (ACA) took hold in 2013. Then we discuss what has happened since 2013 under the ACA with commercial insurance and the problems that remain.

## EMPLOYER-BASED INSURANCE AND HOW IT WORKS: A QUICK HISTORY

Neither long tradition nor well-thought-out public policy is responsible for the fact that much health insurance is arranged at the workplace through employers (so-called *employer-based* insurance). The practice came about during the wage freezes of World War II. By law, employers were not permitted to offer higher wages to attract scarce workers. So, instead, employers began providing free health care to employees and their families as a benefit. The law was written so that health insurance was a "before-tax" business expense. Congress eventually added this benefit to the Internal Revenue Code and made the status of employer-sponsored health insurance permanent, meaning that even today the employer does not pay tax on health-care benefits provided to workers, making it a form of employee compensation. Over time, providing employer-sponsored health benefits became standard in most large US companies.

In 1974, Congress gave employers another break in the Employee Retirement Income Security Act.[5] ERISA, as it's known, governs how private employers, along with pension and insurance companies, administer their benefits. For health care, ERISA applies only to those employers who "self-fund" their insurance—what used to be called *self-insurance*. Employers who self-fund pay all health-care expenses themselves. They use *third-party administrators*—or TPAs, usually a large insurance company—to do the claims processing, send bills, and pay providers.

For self-funded employers, it's largely a myth that insurance companies decide what is and is not paid; actually, it is the employer who decides broadly what to cover. The insurance company, acting as a TPA, simply carries out those wishes. For ERISA plans, there were few health regulations, permitting those employers a great deal of flexibility. About 60 percent of all workers in the United States are in ERISA plans. Almost all larger employers self-fund their plans and thus fall into this category.[6] Why is this important? We know that health-care insurance is regulated by states, but ERISA plans are not. In fact, only about 20 percent of people with health insurance have plans regulated by state law.[7] Therefore changes made by states in health-insurance regulations and laws—such as regulating the price of health insurance—affect only one in five insured.

This was the situation until the ACA came about. The majority of regulations in the ACA were put into the ERISA law, marking the first time ERISA plans had some serious requirements. Self-funded plans now have provisions that eliminate yearly and lifetime maximums—which cap the amount insurance will pay out for care—and that maintain coverage for children up to age twenty-six on a parent's plan, as well as prohibiting exclusion of those with preexisting conditions.

## THE PROS AND CONS OF THE EMPLOYER-BASED SYSTEM

### Pros

Receiving health insurance at work is easy for the employee. The employer simply deducts the employee's share of the health-insurance premium as part of the payroll process. This "automatic" payroll feature of the employer-based insurance system is attractive to employees. In the Texas Medical Center's Health Policy Institute's annual consumer survey, more than twice as many employees said they would rather have their employer arrange insurance coverage than be given money to purchase insurance on their own.[8]

Since health-insurance expenses are excluded from taxable income, the employer is left with considerable savings.[9] This exclusion cost the federal government an estimated $260 billion in income and payroll taxes in 2017.[10] There are tax advantages for employees too, who generally pay about 30 percent of the monthly premium for themselves (and more for a family), with employers picking up the rest. But like employers, employees pay this amount with "pretax" dollars, which allows them to pay less out of pocket. Interestingly, the savings to the employee are usually greater when the employer pays for their insurance than if the employee were paid what the employer spent on their behalf. We have economic incentives that encourage both sides of the equation to support the status quo for employer-sponsored insurance.

## Cons

Despite tax and administrative advantages, employer-based insurance has some negative features, one of which is the enormous cost of health care to businesses. According to the US Bureau of Labor Statistics, employers' average health-care cost per employee has doubled over the last fifteen years.[11] Many employers believe the "hassle" of offering health insurance, which requires hiring internal benefits managers or expensive outside contracting agents, is too costly as well. In addition to the time investment, the costs for billing and enrollment are also significant, particularly for small businesses, where insurance is more expensive.

For almost all businesses, providing health care is not their "core business"; yet many find themselves forced to learn how to effectively negotiate the health-insurance industry in order to obtain the best price in quality health care. Essentially, most employers must be in the business of health care even if they aren't experts. Some become important change agents. For example, the Leapfrog Group, a collection of more than two hundred employers that purchases health care for more than thirty-seven million people in the United States, has provided leadership in using the employer-based health-insurance system to require certain quality standards, such as insisting that hospitals provide round-the-clock coverage of intensive-care units by physicians.[12] In an ideal world, any businesses should not need to provide stimuli for health-system change. The health systems should define and deliver the highest-quality care. But the world isn't that kind of ideal.

Finally, before the ACA was enacted, our system of employer-provided health insurance forced "job lock," meaning that if an employee had a chronic condition such as diabetes or cancer, the insurance company could refuse to insure that specific disease or refuse to cover the person at all. This was called the *preexisting-condition exclusion*. Employees with health conditions who wanted to switch jobs or leave their employer to start their own business were often reluctant to do so, fearing loss of health-insurance coverage by the new employer due to a preexisting-condition exclusion. For the time being, this is not an issue, as the ACA prohibits preexisting condition exclusions. In 2017, but for one vote in the Senate, preexisting-condition exclusions would have been reintroduced.[13] Never say never.

## NOT ALL BUSINESSES ARE CREATED EQUAL

There are about 7.4 million employers in the United States, 1.4 million of which have more than two hundred employees, and virtually all of those offer health insurance to their workers.[14]

But most businesses, about 60 percent, are small businesses with fewer than ten workers, and less than half of them offer health insurance.[15] The primary reason they decline to provide coverage is cost. For small businesses, the cost of providing health insurance is higher than it is for larger businesses for several reasons.

1. Administrative costs to the insurance company for small businesses may be up to 40 percent greater per employee than for large businesses. Small businesses are more likely than large firms to be in the goods and services labor sectors, such as construction, restaurants, agriculture, and fishing. These labor sectors report higher percentages of employees that work part-time, and with higher turnover, which requires more frequent changes in the updating of employee information, which, in turn, increases costs for the company.

2. Three-quarters of work-related injuries occur in the goods and services sector (such as burns in restaurants), thus making their health-care costs and premiums higher.

3. Because health insurance is more expensive for employers and workers in small businesses, the workers who do purchase insurance may do so because they have greater health needs, leading to *adverse selection*, an important concept of insurance that directly relates to the ability to spread risk over a large number of employees. If only those who are sick buy insurance, the cost of premiums increases because there are fewer well people to pay for the costs of the sick members. And when fewer and fewer well people sign up for insurance, an *insurance death spiral* can result, leaving insurance companies to cover more and more sick people with fewer dollars from well people paying into the system, spiraling up the cost of insurance. And with few takers, the insurance company withdraws coverage altogether.

4. A single small business with few employees has less clout to negotiate health-insurance-premium rates, compared to a large business. Because of the higher expense, a small business is also able to offer less choice of plans. Seventy percent of businesses with fewer than two

hundred employees offered just one plan; compare this number to 80 percent of those companies with more than two hundred employees that were able to offer at least two choices. Having less choice in plans usually means that the single plan in a market can have relatively high prices. The unavailability of a lower-cost alternative means that young, healthy, or low-income workers may find the single-option employer-sponsored coverage too costly and may choose not to buy coverage at all.

If small businesses provide health insurance at all, they provide fewer choices at rates that are 8–18 percent higher than those of larger businesses.[16] Frequently the employer requires the employee to pay as much as 50 percent of the premium.[17]

## THE NONGROUP INSURANCE MARKET

Before the Affordable Care Act was fully enacted in 2013, the only way to obtain health coverage for any person whose employer did not offer insurance and who was not eligible for group or public health insurance like Medicare or Medicaid was in the individual or *nongroup* insurance market—which refers to the fact that these people buy insurance on their own and not as part of a group of employees. Consumers would go to an insurance broker and purchase a plan for themselves or their family, just like they'd buy automobile insurance. In 2013, about 4 percent of the US population purchased health insurance in the nongroup market.[18] Nongroup insurance premiums have varied more than group premiums paid by large businesses, and generally the coverage was less adequate.

To better understand how working Americans dealt with the nongroup health-insurance market before the Affordable Care Act took effect, let's consider a family of four: The parents are in their midthirties, and no one in the family has had any unusual health-care expenses. In 2013, the average premium for this family was $5,088, and every year, before insurance would begin to help paying their medical-care costs, the family had to pay a deductible of $4,178, for a total of $9,266 out-of-pocket spending.[19] Let's also assume that both parents work in a local small business, such as a restaurant or dry cleaner not offering health insurance, and are paid minimum wage at $7.25 per hour, making a combined income of $30,160 per year. Because the federal poverty level for a family of four was $23,550 in 2013, this family would have earned too much for their children to be covered by Medicaid. And remember, since this was 2013, there weren't yet any market exchanges where the family could get subsidies to buy insurance. So they were on their own to pay a minimum of $9,266 in premiums and deductibles when they bring home only $30,160 before taxes. That's 31 percent of their income.

## HOW MUCH CAN PEOPLE AFFORD?

What, we might ask, is "reasonable" to expect a family to pay for health care as a percentage of income? Budgeting websites suggest a family of four earning $30,000 per year would have $400 to $800 left to pay for everything else—after paying rent, utilities, food, transportation, childcare, Internet access, and income tax. "Health care" fits in that "everything else" category. Actually, no, it doesn't "fit."

It is no wonder people are uninsured: they can't afford to pay for it. [20]

So, is health care affordable? Let's consider the answer in terms of a percentage of a family's income. Some experts suggest for low-income families earning below about $30,000 that 2–5 percent is the most that's really affordable to spend on health care. [21] To find out whether that's correct, we surveyed nine thousand consumers nationally. [22] Virtually everyone answered that they considered health insurance to be important, and the overwhelming reason a person lacked insurance was cost. We asked respondents what percentage of their income they would consider an "affordable" amount to spend on health insurance, including premiums, deductibles, and other out-of-pocket costs. Interestingly, both the uninsured and the insured said 2 percent was about right. [23] Of course, many people who had health insurance spent far more than that, but that did not mean they could afford it.

Critics of the uninsured suggest that they could give up frivolous spending ("like flat-screen TVs") to afford their health-care expenses, but half of our respondents said they had already cut back on savings, clothing, and food just to pay for their health care. These survey results likely come as no surprise to you, given that most Americans have less than $1,000 in their savings accounts. [24]

The bottom line is that health insurance and health care are just too expensive, whether a person is working or not, unless the employer foots most of the bill. How do we fix this? We must reduce the price of health care. [25]

## THE EMPLOYER-BASED INSURANCE MARKET SINCE 2013

Several important ACA provisions affected employer-based insurance:[26]

1. With the ACA, the preexisting-condition exclusion was no longer permitted. Furthermore, insurers were not permitted to consider a person's health in setting premiums. Before Obamacare, if an employee had a chronic condition, such as heart disease or cancer, the insurance company could refuse to insure that specific disease or refuse to cover the person at all—limiting the coverage with a preexisting-condition exclusion. There were other ways the insurer could restrict access, like requiring a waiting period after hire (such as three to twelve months) before insurance would go into effect or charging significantly higher premiums for that person. If you developed cancer while you were insured, you'd stay covered. But if you waited until after your diagnosis before seeking insurance, it was often too late to find coverage. The ACA eliminated the exclusion, which meant people—especially those purchasing plans on the individual market—are not rendered uninsurable simply because they have a health condition.

2. It might have seemed cruel, but the preexisting-condition exclusion was really the only way that insurers could "nudge" healthy people to buy insurance. Otherwise patients could save money by refusing to pay for health insurance until they needed it—literally applying for insurance on the way into the hospital for surgery. And if we all did that, insurance simply wouldn't work, with coverage costs spiraling out of control. In the absence of the preexisting-condition exclusion, some stimulus would be necessary to prompt individuals to buy health insurance rather than waiting until they need it. The ACA had a "weak" mandate forcing people to buy health insurance or pay a penalty up to 2 percent of income. Congress repealed the mandate in 2017. Now with no preexisting-condition exclusion and no mandate to buy health insurance, healthy people have no reason to buy insurance, and it seems likely that insurance rates will continue to climb.

3. The ACA allows children up to twenty-six years of age to remain part of a parent's family coverage through an employer. That's the case even if the child isn't a student.

4. The ACA requires health insurers to provide coverage in ten categories of *essential health benefits*: outpatient care, emergency care, hos-

pitalization, maternity and newborn care, mental health and substance use care, prescription drugs, rehabilitation, laboratory services, preventive care (including chronic-disease management), and pediatric services (including dental and vision care). The idea was to ensure that people had a certain minimum level of coverage and help reduce instances in which consumers discovered, in times of great need and much to their surprise, that their insurance covered very little. Many of these plans that covered little were called Association Health Plans, so named because they were created when individuals, small businesses, or associations banded together to create larger pools of customers. *Consumer Reports* said these plans were "so riddled with loopholes, limits, exclusions, and gotchas that [patients] won't come close to covering their expenses if they fall seriously ill."[27] As it turns out, about three million people had insurance plans before the ACA that did not have the ten essential benefits and were therefore not permitted after the ACA went into effect. However, President Obama had told the American people that they would be able to keep their same insurance even after ACA took effect. When this turned out to not be the case, many grew vocally angry, saying the president had not told them the truth, as the plans similar to the Association Health Plans were banned. We speculate that many of these people were healthy, had never used their insurance, and had never even found out what was *not* covered before their plans were declared illegal. These plans have resurfaced and today are being advertised as a solution for the uninsured. These plans currently exclude preexisting conditions, do not cover pregnancy, do not pay for prescription drugs, and have severe limits on what they will pay for hospitalization. The premiums are low—about $150 per month—but the deductibles are out of sight—$12,000 or more.[28] Buyer, beware.

5. The ACA requires employers to provide affordable insurance to their workers, but this requirement only extended to businesses with more than fifty employees. Overwhelmingly, businesses in this category were already providing employees with health insurance, so this mandate was not helpful and resulted in a tremendous amount of effort to file the required forms.[29]

6. The ACA prohibits annual and lifetime limits on what insurance companies pay.

7. From 2012 to 2017, the cost of health insurance for individual employee premiums paid by employers increased 18 percent, while the cost to the employee portion increased 21 percent. For family coverage, employer costs rose just 8 percent, while employee costs rose a striking 46 percent, indicating an increased cost shift toward employees.[30] In 2017, the average individual portion of premium plus deductible in employer-sponsored plans was $9,044. For an individual making $30,000 per year, that's about 30 percent of annual income. For health insurance to be truly affordable, the costs should not exceed 2–5 percent of income (maybe up to 8 percent). For an income of $30,000, $600 to $1,500 per year is affordable, not $9,044.[31]

**What Did the ACA Do?**

It's true that the ACA made huge improvements to coverage for health care in the United States. Importantly, with its passage, insurers can no longer exclude those with preexisting conditions from coverage. The uninsured population has declined from almost 17 percent of nonelderly adults to 10 percent.[32] And there are important minimum standards for what is covered by health insurance. But the law hasn't solved one of the biggest problems facing US health care: Prices are increasing at an unsustainable rate and must be decreased. The ACA had essentially no provisions designed to reduce the cost of health care, and it shows. We will discuss this topic in the following chapters and suggest some solutions.

## CHAPTER SUMMARY

- Kellyanne Conway, senior White House aide to President Trump, believes that if able-bodied people want insurance, they should get a job like she has, and then they'll be covered. But the truth is that 75 percent of people without insurance have at least one full-time worker in their family, and 74 percent of nonelderly uninsured employees work for an employer that does not offer health insurance. Many employers don't offer insurance, and it's even more expensive to get it on your own.
- Today's system of employer-provided insurance wasn't the result of careful, deliberate policy decision-making but is a relic of World War II–era wage freezes, when the government permitted employers to attract workers with health-care benefits.

- More than 90 percent of businesses with more than two hundred employees provide insurance. This puts virtually every large employer in the health-care business, even though they probably don't want to be there.
- In 2017, the average individual portion of premium plus deductible in employer-sponsored plans was $9,044. For an individual making $30,000 per year, that's about 30 percent of annual income. For health insurance to be truly affordable, the costs need to be 2–5 percent of income, which for an income of $30,000 is between $600 and $1,500.
- Between 2012 and 2017, for employer-sponsored insurance, the cost to the employee for single-person coverage increased 21 percent. For family coverage, employee costs rose a striking 46 percent, indicating an increased cost shift toward employees. The ACA's lack of attention to increasing cost has both caused many legislators to try to repeal and provided an opportunity for others to attack costs and work toward the goal of health care for all.

*Chapter Thirteen*

# Myth: The Uninsured Get Adequate Care in the Emergency Department

"I mean, people have access to health care in America," he said. "After all, you just go to an emergency room."[1] Then-president George W. Bush suggested that emergency-room care—the most expensive and least effective way of treating patients with ongoing health conditions—was an appropriate way for treating the uninsured. It also is one of the most common misconceptions people have about health care. While it's true that emergency departments (EDs) don't turn people away in dire situations, the care that EDs provide can hardly be considered adequate for patients with conditions such as cancer, heart failure, and diabetes.

## EMERGENCY DEPARTMENTS MUST SEE ALL PEOPLE

When we talk about a patient having *access* to medical care, what we're talking about is whether that person gets to see a doctor or nurse when the patient thinks they need medical care. By law, anyone who shows up to an emergency department must be seen—so President Bush was technically right. But this was not always the law. In the 1980s, some EDs were refusing to treat low-income patients. After undergoing what was known as the *wallet biopsy*, if the patient seeking treatment failed to show an ability to pay for treatment, they'd be sent off to another hospital. Many times these transfers occurred while the patient was having an emergency such as a heart attack or active labor. In 1986, Congress passed the Emergency Medical Treatment and Labor Act—known as the EMTALA for short, or the "antidumping statute"—mandating that any time a patient arrives at an ED, the hospital must (1) perform an examination to see whether an emergency exists, (2) provide necessary treatment when an emergency does exist, and (3) stabilize the patient and only transfer the patient to another hospital if more advanced care is needed that this second hospital can provide.[2]

## BOTH THE UNINSURED AND THE INSURED OVERUSE THE EMERGENCY DEPARTMENT

It is easy to see why the uninsured, who have nowhere else to go for medical care, use the ED. As we discussed in previous chapters, in many cases there is no true safety net to catch the uninsured when they require medical care.[3] Our problem isn't just that the uninsured overuse the ED; it's that the uninsured and the insured *both* overuse the ED.[4] A number of different studies show that between 37 and 71 percent of visits to emergency departments are by patients who do not have a medical emergency.[5] The range is so wide due to people's different definitions of *emergency*. But even according to the lower end of the estimate, more than a third of patients sitting in the ED don't really need to be there. About half of ED patients arrived at night or on the weekend—slightly more for the uninsured. Meanwhile, about 19 percent of insured patients were admitted, versus 15 percent of uninsured. That suggests only slightly more of the uninsureds' ED visits are elective.[6]

Why are we so concerned with the number of people using the ED? With increased numbers of people waiting in an ED, problems arise. For example, crowding leads to the spread of infectious diseases. In one study, patients admitted to the hospital from a crowded ED had a 5 percent higher mortality in the hospital than those from less crowded EDs.[7] Another danger is that the patients who do not have a true emergency crowd out those who do. When ED rooms become full, and a large number of patients are still waiting for care, a hospital may declare a *diversion*, in which the ED accepts no new patients and arriving ambulances are sent away to other hospitals. Ambulance diversion occurs roughly five hundred thousand times per year, or about once every minute. Not surprisingly, if a hospital is on diversion, ambulances have to travel longer distances. One study found heart attack patients were more likely to die if their closest hospital was on diversion.[8] The Institute of Medicine declared EDs "at the breaking point" several years ago, for good reason.[9]

It's unfair to blame this type of crowding only on the uninsured. They do overuse the ED, but so do insured people. It's important for us to acknowledge this fact, because policy makers need to take steps to discourage both types of patients from unnecessary ED visits. If they only target the uninsured, they won't address the entire problem of overuse.

Another study highlighted by *Vox* sheds light on the situation. In 2013, about 12.2 of uninsured people visited the ED, compared to 11.1 percent of privately insured people—in other words, in roughly equal amounts. However, we see a stark difference in another area: While 76.7 percent of privately insured people had an outpatient or primary-care visit that year, only 41.8 percent of uninsured people did. "The problem is not so much that the uninsured go to the emergency room more than other people," Zhou and colleagues wrote in *Health Affairs*. "The problem might be instead that they don't get other kinds of care as often."[10]

## DO THE UNINSURED GET ALL THE CARE THEY NEED IN THE EMERGENCY DEPARTMENT?

The uninsured definitely don't get all the care they need at the ED. The difference between the insured and uninsured, as we have seen above, is that the uninsured may have no other place to go and therefore rely on the ED by default to provide all their care. Regular preventive care such as blood pressure measurement, cholesterol checks, cancer screenings, and the necessary follow-up just aren't done in the ED.[11] *Of course they take your blood pressure in the ED*, you might insist. But to truly diagnose hypertension, three visits showing an abnormal reading are necessary—which doesn't happen in the ED. As we've stated before, uninsured people between the ages of nineteen and sixty-four die at a rate 40 percent higher than those with health insurance.[12] Clearly the uninsured don't get the care they need.[13] If they did, those figures wouldn't be so stark, and uninsured wouldn't be arriving in EDs in advanced stages of disease like heart failure, cancer, or untreated severe psychiatric illness. But they are.[14] When they are admitted to the hospital after an ED visit, the uninsured have to stay longer and have higher mortality rates than the insured, indicating that they arrived in worse condition.[15] And the uninsured leave the hospital against medical advice more than three times as often as the insured.[16]

# WHAT CAN BE DONE?

Important changes are necessary to make sure the uninsured have access to medical care and also to make sure that scarce resources are available to treat true medical emergencies in emergency departments. In a number of areas, clinics have extended night and weekend availability of physicians to treat nonemergent cases. Or perhaps patients with minor illnesses could be cared for in the ED but by nurses or paraprofessionals who would "line them up" for the physician to see quickly—a practice now done with medical students that could become standard practice in all EDs.

Another way of reducing ED use among the insured would be for health-insurance companies to make wider use of "triage" phone lines or video calls that patients can use to find out whether their condition is a real emergency or if it's safe to wait to address the medical issue until they can get an appointment with a health-care provider. In the Grand-Aides program, a nurse can dispatch a nurse's aide to make a home visit and send video back to the nurse supervisor. One study in Denver, for example, found that about two-thirds of the time that parents felt their child needed to go to the ED, an emergency visit wasn't really medically necessary.[17] In line with this work, a study of children receiving Medicaid benefits found that better using Grand-Aides and nurse supervisors could have reduced ED visits by 74 percent.[18]

For the uninsured, hospitals themselves could make triage phone lines available, since ostensibly, subsidizing the costs of staffing them would be far less than providing uncompensated care. More important, we need to expand the safety net—which in many cases is nonexistent—to ensure the uninsured have other options to see doctors besides showing up at the ED.

Some insurers are seeking to penalize patients for seeking nonemergent care in emergency departments, requiring patients to pay out of pocket if it is determined that they didn't have a true medical emergency.[19] This practice could be made more "patient friendly" if the insurer were to waive the ED charge if the patient called the insurer nurse line and the nurse recommended going to the ED.

In short, it's a grim picture for the uninsured. They are sicker when they arrived at the ED, and they leave the hospital against medical advice more often than the insured, with an increased likelihood of death in the hospital. It's no wonder our life expectancy compared to other countries is so short. What President Bush said is partially true: The uninsured have access to some care in the ED. But for a large segment of our population, this care is not enough.

Martin Luther King Jr. put it best: "Of all the forms of inequality, injustice in health care is the most shocking and inhumane."[20]

## CHAPTER SUMMARY

- Even former presidents think the ED can provide appropriate access to care.
- In 1986, to combat the increasing numbers of emergency departments turning away uninsured patients in an emergency—including active labor—Congress passed the Emergency Medical Treatment and Labor Act, requiring ED to assess all patients and provide emergency treatment.
- This law permitted uninsured patients—and also insured patients—to use the ED as a clinic. Studies estimate that about 50 percent of ED patients don't have a true medical emergency. These people crowd EDs sufficiently that about half million times each year EDs declare diversions, where ambulances are turned away. Heart attack patients whose nearest hospitals had high levels of diversion were more likely to die.
- The uninsured arrive in the EDs in advanced stages of disease like heart failure, cancer, or untreated severe psychiatric illness. When they are admitted, the uninsured have increased length of stay and greater mortality during hospitalization than the insured. And the uninsured leave the hospital against medical advice more than three times as often as the insured.
- What can be done? We can address overuse of EDs by keeping more clinics open 24/7 and, in those places where patients do not have access to these clinics, using nurses or paraprofessionals to see patients with non-emergent conditions to prepare them for quick treatment by a physician. We can also set up nurse call lines, permitting insurance companies to decrease unnecessary ED visits. We can likewise help address the uninsured who overuse EDs by steering them to FQHCs and other primary-care providers.

*Chapter Fourteen*

# Myth: The Market Can Fix Health Care

Members of Congress and newspaper opinion writers alike want to "Get government out and let markets work in health care."[1] For reasons we'll outline later in this chapter, that probably won't ever be possible—and we'll discuss why that might not even be a goal we should strive for. We'll tell you up front that patients will never know as much as doctors, and so *information asymmetry* will always exist. That doesn't mean that we should not work on price transparency, making information available to consumers so they can understand it, and other improvements that the US medical-care system well needs. It's just that simply saying "Let the market do it" doesn't work and won't actually fix the system's problems.

Let's first try to understand a few basic principles about what a *market* is.

## WHAT IS A MARKET?

Whether it's an exchange for buying oranges or paying for health care, the ten principles of a market are the same. Professor Sandra Schickele has created an extremely helpful way to look at the characteristics of a market:

1. In every market, there is *perfect information*, meaning that buyers and sellers both have all the necessary information about a product or service, including price. Importantly, they all have the same information, and they understand the information equally well.
2. There is *perfect competition*, in that each product or service is the same, no matter who produces it, and they're all priced the same. The

higher the price, the more willing a seller will by to *supply* it; the higher the price, the less willing a buyer will be to *demand* it.

3. Production has no *barriers to entry*—meaning anyone can make the product—and there is no lag time in making the product. Money and labor can move from one producer to another without anything getting in the way.
4. The deal between a specific seller and a specific buyer does not affect anyone else.
5. There are no *free riders*. In other words, nobody gets the product or service unless they pay for it.
6. There is no *dependence* on others—meaning no seller depends on another seller to produce their product.
7. There are no *economies of scale*, which means that there is no discount for producing or buying or selling in bulk: it costs the same to make one product as to make one thousand.
8. The smallest product is the right size for even the smallest buyer. For example, soft drinks used to be available only in twelve-ounce cans. Recently, the 7.5-ounce can has been introduced as customers told manufacturers that they wanted less soda per can.
9. The costs of making the deal are included in the price.
10. There is little to no government intervention. [2]

Before you read further, please go back up to the list and think about whether you can come up with any examples in the current US health-care system that don't fit within the definition of a market. We have already acknowledged that in health care there will always be information asymmetry between the doctor, who has studied and then practiced the specialized subject for years, and the patient, who necessarily knows considerably less about medicine. But, in actuality, the US health-care system does not meet *any one* of the above criteria for being a market, meaning US health care is clearly *not* a market. Let's explore this a little more deeply.

## CHARACTERISTICS OF HEALTH CARE INCONSISTENT WITH A MARKET

1. The most glaring example of how US health care fails to meet the standard of a market is the lack of *perfect information* in health care. Unless all patients and their physicians have the same information,

and the same understanding of that information, we don't have perfect information. Instead, we have *information asymmetry*, and to a certain extent, this will always exist between physicians and their patients. When your doctor tells you that you really need to undergo a certain test, chances are that you will take their advice. Unless you went to medical school, you likely have no way of evaluating whether that test is truly necessary to ensuring your health or being performed for some other reason. Recently there's been renewed attention to the fact that drug manufacturers do not allow pharmacists, to whom they sell their drugs, to advise patients of the cheapest way to buy their prescription.[3] In many cases, an insured patient could save money on drugs if paying in cash and not using insurance, but pharmacists can't and don't disclose that information.

2. Another clear example of health care being far from a pure market is its lack of *perfect competition*. In a world of perfect competition, all surgeons would have the same results. But they don't, and we can't even compare with certainty their results on even similar patients. In perfect competition, all MRI tests would be priced the same. They aren't, and we are not sure what all the varying prices are. An interesting issue is that, in some cases, people not only are willing but actually prefer to spend more on expensive care because they think it must be better. Certainly this is the opposite of how a market should behave.[4]

## Moral Hazard

Another issue that gets us far away from perfect competition occurs when people who have health insurance don't worry as much about the cost of the procedure or test. *Moral hazard* is the willingness to assume risk because you know somebody else is going to protect you from all of the consequences of your risky actions.[5] In the case of health insurance, as long as the insurance company pays for the patient's care, the patient is shielded from the high cost of their health care. This means that insured patients and families are not as affected by the high cost of medical care. In high-deductible health plans, the patient must pay a significant amount before insurance begins to pay, the theory being that patients will be careful about how they spend their own money. But patients do not always choose wisely, and they are largely unaffected by costs—or at least not as greatly—once they've met their deductible and insurance pays for most of their medical care.

## Physician-Induced Demand

Certain unique circumstances make it even less likely that the US health-care system could ever be a market. This concerns the ways that both physicians and patients increase the demand for medical care. On one hand, we have *physician-induced demand* for medical care, in which the physician recommends that the patient receive the very service the physician is paid to perform. Consider this familiar scenario: an auto mechanic is incentivized to sell you that tune-up and says your engine just doesn't sound right to him. But in the case of health care, the stakes are much higher. What about the spine surgeon who recommends, based on his diagnosis, that the patient hire him to perform spine surgery? With the information asymmetry pervasive in health care, patients generally follow their physician's recommendations. Plenty of data exist demonstrating physician-induced demand. It has been found, for example, that obstetricians perform 10 percent fewer caesarian sections when they know the patient is a physician or nurse. At least one possibility is that the OB knows they can't get away with performing an unnecessary procedure on a colleague.[6] A more subtle example is when a physician orders tests that do not provide direct financial benefit, but the lab running the tests is owned by the physician. This is illegal. But what if the owner of the lab and the physician frequently have dinner together, and the owner always picks up the entire tab? That's also illegal but surely more difficult to track.

## Patient-Induced Demand

We also see *patient-induced demand* when patients seek—or demand—medical care that isn't really necessary. Some examples include the parent who brings a child to the emergency department for a cold or the patient who requests a new drug from their physician based entirely on advertising directed toward consumers. One study found that primary-care physicians prescribe the drug requested by the patient 77 percent of the time as long as it won't hurt the patient—just to shorten the visit.[7]

Briefly, let's discuss some of the other characteristics of health care that prevent it from being a true market:

3. There are no barriers to entry in a true market, but that can't be said for health care. How about medical school and nursing school? Those are pretty high "barriers to entry." Physicians also put up barriers that prevent nurse practitioners from being able to practice medicine with-

out a doctor's supervision, despite data showing that the nurse practitioners have similar results as physicians. That's another big one. You get the idea.

4. In a true market, there are no effects on anyone (e.g., a third party) except the seller and the buyer. For small employers who provide health insurance to their employees, the high cost of just one patient can wind up increasing health care costs for all employees. In some cases, the impact can even extend to larger groups. A famous example is the Iowa teenager whose hemophilia treatment cost $1 million per month in medical bills. The case grew widespread attention since his insurer, Wellmark Blue Cross and Blue Shield, said the teenager's medical care was so expensive that it contributed to rising premiums for thousands of other Iowa customers.[8]

5. The market does not allow *free riders*—which means that no one gets the product if they don't pay for it. Of course, we have a government-sponsored system that provides health care to those who can't afford to pay for it, called Medicaid. Meanwhile, in emergencies, hospitals are required to stabilize patients even if they lack the ability to pay for treatment.

6. True markets do not allow for dependence on others, meaning one seller cannot depend on another seller to produce their product. Yet a surgeon requires an anesthesiologist, and both of them require a hospital. Each "seller" in the health-care system is closely linked to many others.

7. There are no economies of scale in a true market, which means the cost for additional products is the same as for one product. But that's not the case for health care. For example, large employers pay lower prices for health insurance than small employers do; the big companies are able to negotiate for better terms since they're bringing the insurance companies so many customers. Similarly, large health insurers have the clout to negotiate for better payment rates with health-care providers.

8. The smallest product is the right size for even the smallest buyer in a true market. But in health care, any one particular physician is capable of caring for approximately three thousand patients; this means that the physician will not locate to a town that has only one thousand patients, as the "product"—the physician's services—is too large for the "buyer"—the small town without enough potential patients.

9. In a true market, the costs of making the deal are included in the price. However, if a physician decides to make a house call, they cannot bill for the transportation time.

10. There is little to no government intervention in a true market. That can hardly be said of the US health-care system.

There are numerous ways in which the government "intervenes" in health care:

1. *As a payer.* About half of people with health insurance are covered by government programs such as Medicare and Medicaid.[9] It is unlikely that the government will stop paying for these programs altogether; however, in the Trump administration, we have an example of the government getting to decide who is covered by Medicare and Medicaid and how much they will pay for care. The American Health Care Act of 2017—which passed in the House and came within one vote of passing in the Senate—would have reduced Medicaid funding by close to $900 billion, which would essentially have rolled back Medicaid expansion across the United States, taking health care away from twenty million people. The Texas Medical Center's survey shows that 90 percent of respondents were against this intervention.[10] It is clear that, as payers, we want to continue to see at least the current level of government involvement in our health care.

2. *As a benchmark.* The vast majority of those over sixty-five years old are covered by Medicare. Not only does Medicare set prices for how much it pays physicians and hospitals for the people covered by Medicare, but these prices also become the baseline for how private insurers pay. Groups of physicians decide the *relative value* of tests and procedures. For example, physicians decide that coronary bypass surgery is worth fifty units, and reading an electrocardiogram about 0.5 units. Medicare pays $38 per unit. That would mean a physician would be reimbursed $1,900 for bypass surgery and $19 for the ECG. Insurers then decide what they will pay based on multiple Medicare rates.

3. *Deciding what to pay for.* Many a legislator has accused the government of standing between patients and physicians every time the government withholds payment for medical care. But it turns out that, in actuality, Medicare pays for pretty much anything that is not experimental; in fact, the government intervenes less than commercial insur-

ers. In one case, McAllen, Texas, was singled out for having the second-highest cost of health care in the United States.[11] But it turned out that the data used was for Medicare patients. And when McAllen was analyzed for costs borne by insurance companies, the data showed that McAllen's expenditures were right on par with costs in the rest of the United States. In other words, the government was much more lenient—it intervened less—than the insurance companies.[12]

4. *Regulating sales of insurance across state lines.* Some have called for "opening up the market" by allowing for the sale of insurance across state lines.[13] While it seems attractive to "open the borders" and allow for people, in the individual nongroup market, to buy insurance in another state, the predictions do not point toward lower premiums. Actually, the opposite is likely to happen. In that case, individuals would be permitted to buy insurance in any state that permits skimpy benefits and has *benefit riders* that exclude certain diseases (sound like preexisting conditions?). Healthy people would buy insurance in those states, leaving behind all of the sick people in their state. Also, in order for an insurer to provide access to physicians, nurses, and hospitals in the new state, the insurers would have to start from scratch with providers in that state. Surely the new insurer would need to pay more than existing insurers (or why would the physicians sign up with patients from the new insurer?), resulting in higher premiums for the newcomers. Finally, the patient would have to go to that state for care unless the practitioners were licensed in the patient's state of residence. So, it's not really clear how "opening up the market" will reduce any price.

## WILL HEALTH CARE EVER
## SATISFY THE CONDITIONS OF A MARKET?

We have seen that the US health-care system fails to fit every single market criterion. While some of these conditions may change (and it is not clear that many of them need to change), it's likely impossible that US health care could ever satisfy all the conditions of a market.

## Can Information and Competition Be Improved Sufficiently to Have Health Care Act More "Market-Like?"

Harvard Business School professors Michael E. Porter and Elizabeth Teisberg, who run the Value Institute for Health & Care, describe a utopia where "competition occurs in prevention, diagnosis, and treatment of health conditions" and where "consumers of health care would get the information they need to make decisions about care."[14] But there are numerous barriers standing in the way.

Ideally consumers should be able to see clear data on *outcomes*—or what sort of success or failure their health-care provider has when treating any given condition. But how do we presently decide who gets "credited" with a patient death? In most instances, the surgeon has the mortality counted against them, even if the hospitalist wrote the prescription on discharge for the drug that had a rare side effect in the patient. For this reason, physicians fight against having data reported at the level of the physician and would instead prefer to see it reported for the whole health system. Current dogma in the medical sector is that we should never place blame on individuals, especially given all the shades of gray. But this concept hides the single repetitive bad actor.

Second, it's not totally clear that patients actually *want* to sift through quality data. Patients may be too busy, or too sick, to look up the data, even when data are available. And third, these data are not, in general, presented in a way that patients can understand.

A great starting place is the "plain-language" initiative taken by the Texas insurance commissioner, where eventually all insurance documents will be written in language understandable to the average patient, rewording "letters and forms with an eye toward shorter words and formats that are easier to read."[15]

## What Is the Appropriate Role of Government in Health Care?

It is impossible to eliminate government involvement in health care entirely, nor should we want to (for example, we don't want to get rid of Medicare). Health care in the United States, therefore, cannot ever be a true market. The question of how much government is tolerable will, to a certain extent, depend on how one views the role of government. However, it's important to acknowledge that where there is true "market failure"—in other words, where the market isn't working—some government intervention is almost always required.

Let's go back and examine the ten characteristics of a market and see how different players might help the market failures that exist. We suggest government intervention only as the last resort in the case of market failure.[16]

1. *Perfect information.* Remember, about 5 percent of people use health information in decision-making, and most don't understand it. There are a lot of ways that this problem can be attacked. Surely it is to the insurer's benefit for patients to act wisely when making decisions about how to spend money on health care. Some organization would gather and then publish the best practices on the use of quality information. Perhaps the National Academy of Medicine could perform this function[17]—or a number of nonprofit organizations that absolutely cannot bow to political pressure. Hereafter we'll refer to this unbiased body as "an organization" (though it need not all be the same organization addressing every problem).

2. *Perfect competition.* We surely don't want to eliminate competition in health care, as it is one of the best ways to stimulate improvement. An organization needs to help with publishing prices that can be compared among different providers. Those with high-deductible health plans could be a "proving ground" for how well the information is displayed and used.

3. *No barriers to entry.* Repayment of loans required to pay for medical school (or even college) is a barrier to entry for those who want to become rural primary-care physicians. PCPs, as they are known, often leave medical school with incredibly high loans, and the income as a rural PCP may not be sufficient to repay them. And for some, career choice among physicians is dependent on the amount of loans the physician has to repay.[18] The government may support programs that repay student loans.[19] The government could be the council of a small town that needs a physician. The council could pay for medical- or nursing-school tuition in return for five years of medical service in that town. Many states have such programs—as does the federal government, in the National Health Service Corps. The financial support these programs provide seems to fall when federal or state budgets are tight. In fact, these programs should be increased in tough times or areas of demonstrated shortage.

4. *No effects on anyone (e.g., a third party) except the seller and the buyer.* The government does not have a large role in insurance pricing unless the government is paying for the care. It does set a minimum in Medicaid.

5. *No free riders.* A free rider gets the product whether or not they pay for it. If the government is going to pay for care for those with low income—as they do for Medicaid recipients, for example—they will of necessity be creating free riders, or people getting services even if they don't pay for them. In this case, *free rider* shouldn't have a negative connotation; it's important that those who cannot afford health care nevertheless have a mechanism to obtain it.

6. *No dependence on others.* Dependence occurs where one seller depends on another seller to produce their product. In fact, we want team care—a system where a group of health-care workers cooperate to provide the best care possible for a patient. An organization could work with all sectors to improve how care is delivered with teams.

7. *No economies of scale.* With no economies of scale, the cost for additional products is the same as for one product. An organization could be certain that the true cost of a test or procedure is known and displayed. If larger employers have economies of scale, this information should be made available in ways understandable to members of the public.

8. *The smallest product is the right size for even the smallest buyer.* Let's say that a small town has one thousand patients—not enough for a physician to relocate there. This is a problem that is not directly caused or alleviated by government; however, states and the federal government could develop the regulations that would make telemedicine much simpler and less costly.

9. *The costs of making the deal are included in the price.* Government could help to change definitions and payment for some services with "indirect" time, such as travel.

10. *Little to no government intervention.* In this section we have discussed ways where government, or another entity, could intervene appropriately, as a number of these issues are considered "market failures."

## THE BOTTOM LINE: WILL HEALTH CARE EVER SATISFY THE CONDITIONS OF A MARKET?

No, and neither were pigs meant to fly. The concept is flawed: trying to make US health care a market is trying to fit a square peg into a round hole. While following "market-like" conditions might make sense in some circumstances, health care doesn't *need* to be a market, and it never will be. We want to set goals for our health-care system and the delivery of care that are independent of the need to satisfy a market. We cover this topic in the following chapters.

## CHAPTER SUMMARY

- Economists propose ten characterizes of any true market, which, if considered carefully, fail to match our health-care system entirely.

  1. *Perfect information.* Buyers and sellers have all the relevant information on their product.
  2. *Perfect competition.* The products are not different from one another, and have only one price.
  3. *No barriers to entry.* Anyone can make the product.
  4. *The deal between this seller and this buyer does not affect anyone else.*
  5. *No free riders.* A free rider gets the product whether or not he or she pays for it.
  6. *No dependence on others.* Dependence is where one seller depends on another seller.
  7. *No economies of scale.* With no economies of scale, the cost to make additional products is the same.
  8. *The smallest product is the right size for even the smallest buyer.*
  9. *The costs of making the deal are included in the price.*
  10. *Little to no government intervention.*

- Two characteristics of health care will always prevent its being a market:

  1. *The lack of perfect information.* Doctors are always going to know more than patients, meaning that in health care there will always be "information asymmetry."

2. *The lack of perfect competition.* Perfect competition assumes every physician's results are the same; they are not. Additional barriers to perfect competition are moral hazard, where insurers shield the patients from true expense; "physician-induced demand," where the doctor who recommends a service is the same one who benefits financially from performing it; and patient-induced demand, in which if the patient wants a service, they usually get it, regardless of true medical need.

- It's impractical to think the health-care system will ever be set up as a true market. We can make it more market-like, but "leaving it to the market" is just not a reasonable goal.

*Chapter Fifteen*

# Myth: Doctors and Hospitals Should Be Paid Separately for Each Service They Perform

Arthur Garson Sr. manufactured clothing. The workers in his factory were paid a *piece rate*: for every piece of clothing sewn properly, the worker received a bonus. And, not surprisingly, the workers (and Garson's company) sold as much clothing as they could make. His son, this book's coauthor, was paid *fee-for-service* as a pediatric cardiologist: for every heart catheterization he did, he got paid. Like a factory producing clothing, pediatric cardiologists and the hospital catheterization laboratory "sold" as much as they possibly could, and they got paid every time.

When asked about treatment choices, parents routinely told Garson or other physicians, "Do whatever you recommend." That's a big problem. Those instructions are similar to saying, *Whatever you want to sell me, I'll buy*. It's the stuff of dreams to any salesman.

While physicians and hospitals absolutely do have the welfare of the patient in mind, money does drive behavior and, unfortunately, plays a role in the way they approach care. What can we do about it? First, let's briefly review how physicians and hospitals are paid, as well as a bit of how we got here. We'll use Medicare as an example, but virtually every commercial insurance company and Medicaid operate in a similar way.

PHYSICIAN AND HOSPITAL ORGANIZATION AND PAYMENT

## Medicare from 1965 through the Early 1990s

When Medicare was enacted by Congress in 1965, hospitals were paid on a *cost* basis: whatever the hospitals said their costs were, they were paid. "Costs" continued to increase through the years more quickly than inflation, and Medicare continued to pay. In the early 1980s, Medicare developed a payment mechanism called *diagnosis-related groups*—DRGs—in which the hospital was paid for a patient's principal diagnosis regardless of how long the patient was admitted and no matter how much money was spent on the patient, with a few exceptions. For example, the hospital was paid a set amount for a patient with a heart attack. It was not difficult to predict that, under the new system, patients' stays would become shorter. After all, if the hospital got paid the same amount for a long stay as a short stay, the financial incentive would be to keep the stay brief. One study found that typical stays fell from 10.8 days to 7.8 days three years after the new system was enacted. Hospitals were responding to new economic motivators, but, importantly, readmissions did not increase, suggesting that patients were no worse for wear. In other words, the reforms worked as intended: shorter stays saved money without ill effects. [1]

Hospitals and doctors are paid separately. Before 1992, Medicare paid physicians an amount considered "reasonable and customary," as decided by the physician. As the reader can imagine, those charges were sometimes quite high, but they were nonetheless paid. Between 1980 and 1991, national payments for physician services increased from $42 billion to $142 billion. [2] The government decided that a change was needed, so since 1992, Medicare has paid doctors through what's called the *resource-based relative value scale*. RBRVS, as it's called, pays physicians and other medical practitioners for every service they perform—so-called *fee-for service*.

The government told the physician community that there was a certain amount of money available for physician payment under Medicare and that physicians could decide how to dole it out. Each of the approximately nine thousand services doctors perform—from the simplest reading of an electrocardiogram to the most complex surgery—were evaluated by a panel of physicians who decided how many *relative value units*—RVUs—each service deserved. That number provided the basis for determining how much a doctor would be paid for any single service. For example, reading an electrocardiogram was assigned a value of 0.48 RVUs, a physician office visit 2.05, and coronary bypass surgery 63.99.[3] These RVUs translate to Medicare payments of $17.28 for the electrocardiogram, $73.78 for the office visit, and $2,303 for bypass surgery.

The RBRVS is still in use today, and over time the number of physician services performed each year has increased. For example, the amount paid for an outpatients visit is low, and physicians performed more of them. This meant office visits were packed more closely together, and it's why our visits with doctors are a brief eight to fifteen minutes today.[4] This increase in volume to make up for a low price is an example of *behavioral adjustment.* And it's not that different from the behavior seen in the elder Garson's factory: just as his workers knew that they'd get paid more if they could produce more garments in a shift, the doctors understand that they'll get paid more if they can see more patients in a day.

## The 1990s: Health-Maintenance Organizations

Around the same time that RBRVS was changing the payment scheme in health care in the early 1990s, *health-maintenance organizations* were gaining in popularity as another tool in the battle against rising health-care costs. HMOs, as they are more popularly known, were created to provide an *integrated delivery system* to treat patients, in which doctors, hospitals, clinics, and other outpatient services were tied together with a single insurance company. Each patient had a primary-care physician to serve as a "gatekeeper": If a patient wanted to have a visit to a specialist covered by insurance, first the PCP would have to approve referral to the specialist. In the pure *staff HMO* model, physicians were employed by the HMO and were only hired if they agreed to keep referrals and other costs (including hospital admissions) down. The long-term idea was also for patients to have a single electronic health record that allowed for efficient scheduling and sharing of information and that would also offer physicians "decision support," indicating costs of drugs and, in some cases, how to apply practice guidelines (e.g., what sort of treatment to give in specific situations).

The other hallmark of the HMO was that it was paid by *capitation,* meaning the insurance company paid the HMO each month for each person the HMO cared for, regardless of their expenses, for diagnosis and treatment. The amount the HMO was paid was called *per member per month,* or PMPM. In some cases, the HMO paid each physician entirely by capitation, meaning the physician was given a set sum from which to pay for all services for the patient—outpatient visits, procedures, hospitalization, and even the physician's own salary—and was able to keep anything leftover.

In 1993, Dr. Marcia Angell wrote what has become a classic article, hammering the system that had set up "the doctor as double agent," detailing the ways the HMO capitation-payment scheme could pull a physician in opposite directions, pitting the physician's desire to do the right thing for the patient against keeping more money for themselves.[5] Eventually, HMOs stopped paying physicians fixed amounts per patient, instead placing capitation at the level of the entire HMO. For example, instead of giving the physician a set amount per patient for every month the patient was under their care, the HMO leadership would pay doctors again with fee-for-service using RBRVS from the money paid out by the insurance company.

But even with this important change to the capitation-payment scheme, the stimulus remained to do less for the patient, as there was only a certain amount paid, no matter how many services the patient used. There's some debate about the effect of these incentives: It was said at the time that the providers who would undertreat patients due to capitation are the same ones who would end up overtreating patients under a fee-for-service scheme.[6] The number of journal articles finding better care with HMOs is about equal in number to those finding worse care with HMOs.

Nonetheless, the plans to tinker with capitation received blowback from all sides. "A backlash of criticism by doctors, nurses, consumers, and legislators is forcing health plans to abandon a range of cost-cutting practices that reward doctors and hospitals for limiting care," the *New York Times* wrote in 1996.[7] Why did this happen? Several reasons:

1. The insurance and medical communities did not understand or pay enough attention to the public anger directed at HMOs, which were seen to be money-saving tools only. *Managed care* had become synonymous with "less care."
2. The HMO was an integral part of Hillary Clinton's health-care plan; when that eventually fell out of favor, so too did HMOs.
3. Leaders underestimated patients' desire to have more choice of physicians, failing to appreciate the fact that patients vehemently opposed the idea of a gatekeeper that might prevent them from accessing the specialist they wanted.
4. The ability to define and measure quality in the early 1990s was in its infancy. Physicians lacked the tools to measure quality, and as a result

they couldn't prove that quality of care stayed the same even as they cut costs.

5. Capitation required significant changes in both software and people. Those charged with implementing HMOs failed to develop the information infrastructure needed to understand costs and present data in usable form to physicians and administrators. Perhaps more important, physicians were not prepared—intellectually or emotionally—to deal with ordering fewer tests, procedures, and hospital admissions rather than more.

Such was the situation before US health care began to move toward the present model and accountable-care organizations.

## Rising Prices and Physicians Join Hospitals

In the late 1990s and 2000s, small physician groups and solo practitioners found themselves working long hours, scheduling patient visits into increments sometimes as short as eight minutes to make up for the relative decrease in payment for an office visit. One 1996 study showed a primary-care physician allowed patients an average of twenty-three seconds before interrupting to get to the reason for their visit.[8] Then the government began incentivizing physician use of electronic health records. EHRs, it was hoped, would benefit both doctors and patients, allowing for more seamless sharing of records. But EHRs were not yet ready for prime time, and physicians found the process of inputting patient information difficult and time-consuming. That time spent working with EHRs, instead of patients, cost them real money.

The government also appropriately attacked fraud and abuse and then issued regulations to protect patient confidentiality. These initiatives were reasonable but created an administrative nightmare and higher costs relative to the smaller patient populations treated by small physician groups. Physicians became fed up with the administrative work, took down their shingles, and found hospitals willing to employ them.

The hospitals were happy to have the doctors, as the doctors could order all of their patients' tests to be administered in that hospital and its associated clinics and could refer patients to that hospital only. Though this largely remains the state of things today, this arrangement may not endure much longer.

## Physicians and Fee-for-Service

Since 1992, payment for physicians has remained fee-for-service, based on RBRVS. Fee-for-service leads to *physician-induced demand*, where, as we have seen, the physician recommends a service to the patient and then gets paid, incentivizing the physician to continue to recommend more services to more patients. The *information asymmetry*, created because the doctor necessarily knows more about the patient's medical care than the patient, can be lucrative for health-care providers, as patients generally follow their physician's recommendations. It's not unlike the visit to get your oil changed: Suddenly the $35 oil change costs hundreds of dollars more when the mechanic says he sees something concerning under the hood. If you don't know much about cars, you might just shrug and say, "Fix whatever you think needs fixing."

In 2012, Donald Berwick, who ran Medicare and Medicaid for a time under the Obama administration, wrote a landmark article detailing how the United States wastes a third of its health-care dollars—about $1 trillion per year. Of that, about $200 billion is wasted on *overtreatment*, which Berwick defined as "the waste that comes from subjecting patients to care that, according to sound science and the patients' own preferences, cannot possibly help them."[9] The screw tightened when two highly respected physicians, former Senate majority leader Dr. Bill Frist and Dr. Steven Schroeder, declared that "the way physicians are paid drives up medical expenditures."[10] And the evidence continues to mount today. Recently, in a large survey of doctors, more than 70 percent of respondents said doctors "are more likely to perform unnecessary procedures when they profit from them." The study also found that most doctors "believed that de-emphasizing fee-for-service physician compensation would reduce health-care utilization and costs."[11]

Under the influence of the Affordable Care Act, in 2015 Congress enacted the Medicare Access and CHIP Reauthorization Act, which, among other provisions, changed the way the government pays physicians. The idea was to base doctor pay on quality and value, not just the amount of work they do.[12] There are 271 ways these factors are measured, and physicians get to pick which measures they want to be graded on. But physicians have pushed back against the complexity of the program, and many say that it still rewards physicians with fee-for-service payments.

A variety of incentives might prevent physicians from ordering too many tests and performing too many treatments. One suggestion is to pay them salaries and offer bonuses for good performance. And the good news is that many doctors agree this is a great idea. A national survey by our organization, the Texas Medical Center's Health Policy Institute, found that US doctors prefer salaries over the fee-for-service status quo. We found that 69 percent of doctors said their preferred method of compensation would be a high proportion of their pay as straight salary, with a low proportion of their pay based on incentives, or else a straight salary with no incentives at all. [13] Why is this something we consider so important? Because when doctors are paid salaries, they have less incentive to order unnecessary treatment. In fact, moving from fee-for-service to salary has shown savings of 8–33 percent due to a decrease in tests ordered, procedures performed, and hospital admissions. [14]

Some of the best health-care systems in the country salary their physicians, including Mayo Clinic, Cleveland Clinic, and Kaiser Permanente. Other health-care providers would do well to follow their lead.

## Accountable-Care Organizations, Population Health, and Value-Based Care

We now have arrived in our modern history of US health care at 2008, when Barack Obama championed the Affordable Care Act. Signed into law in 2010, the ACA stimulated a new kind of integrated delivery system: the *accountable-care organization*. The ACO, as it is known, had some differences from HMOs, but the idea was the same. The ACO must have a defined population of at least five thousand people. The idea of caring for a specific population was not new—that had surfaced with the HMO.

But now the term *population health* had emerged, along with numerous definitions. According to David Kendig, population health refers to "the health outcomes of a group of individuals, including the 'distribution of such outcomes' within the group." There are two concepts nestled here: (1) *Distribution of outcomes* highlights that *all* members of the population are counted, specifically addressing health disparities, whether due to race or income. In other words, we do not sufficiently understand our population's health outcomes if the only data we have are for the wealthy or only those that show up in the clinic. (2) *Social determinants of health*, as discussed in chapter 1, must be addressed. In practical terms, the ACO may find that some of the ways to address health require more than medical care.

The ACO is rooted in the principle of paying based on *value-based care*—as opposed to paying based on volume. ACOs are permitted to pay fee-for-service but are encouraged to pay for patient management based on value:

1. Pay a bonus, to providers, for meeting certain quality metrics. In other words, if patients do well, so will doctors.
2. Use capitation, also discussed earlier, in which the ACO is paid a certain amount per member, per month, and then decides how it wants to pay physicians and hospitals.
3. Use "bundling" as a way station to capitation, where payment is based on an episode of care for physicians and the hospital. For example, a health-care provider would be paid a flat fee for a hip replacement. Bundling includes absolutely everything associated with a treatment— physician fees, hospital fees, any medications, readmission, or transfer to another hospital or nursing facility for ninety days. Similar to capitation, bundles stimulate physicians and hospitals to do less, since they'd want more money left over at the end of treatment to keep as profit. But bundles come with a downside: they stimulate the ACO to do more bundles (after all, each person has two hips).

Both capitation and bundling put the ACO "at risk" for a patient's care, with a fixed amount of payment regardless of the actual expenses. They do put the incentives in the proper direction not to overdo care, but there is the possibility of doing less than necessary too. Fortunately, today our ability to measure quality of patient care is much better than it was twenty years ago.

This chapter has meant to expose the myth that in a well-functioning health system, doctors and hospitals should be paid for each service they perform. Have you figured out why we call that a myth? Doctors and other providers shouldn't *just* be paid for doing more services, like hip replacements; they aren't the seamstresses at the factory floor. They should be paid for providing value and quality. Ultimately, they shouldn't be paid simply for treating patients. They should be paid for making patients *better* in an efficient manner, which may require working with certain patients to improve their social determinants of health.

Payment method is still a work in progress—or *hopefully* one of progress. The goal is clear: to create a payment system that doesn't stimulate either too many or too few services. The method should also be simple and easy to understand. But providers also must have skin in the game, to allow them to get a bonus for stellar performance or to lose money for subpar performance.

The results of different payment mechanisms must be further studied. We have found numerous methods that don't work. It is time to see what does.

## CHAPTER SUMMARY

- When Medicare and Medicaid were first created in the 1960s, the government paid physicians using a fee-for-service system, paying them for each service performed separately, in whatever amount was deemed "reasonable and customary." Commercial insurers like Blue Cross Blue Shield followed Medicare and Medicaid's lead. This payment method incentivized more procedures, tests, and hospitalizations.
- Fee-for-service payment models lead to overtreatment, costing the United States an estimated at $200 billion per year.
- The federal government began paying hospitals by the patient's diagnosis-related group—DRG—rather than by the number of days hospitalized, resulting in shorter hospitalizations, as hospitals were paid the same amount for long stays as they were for short stays.
- Physician payment was made more "objective" by the resource-based relative value scale, in which each service a physician did was "graded" largely by the amount of effort required. When outpatient visits were given an extremely low score—and, hence, a correspondingly low reimbursement for physicians—physicians made up for the financial shortfall by increasing the number of patients they saw in a day, leading to the rapid pace of visits we see today, or "the eight-minute doctor visit."
- To reduce overtreatment, the Centers for Medicare and Medicaid has committed to *value-based* payment, where the goal is to encourage quality care rather than quantity of care. This transition hasn't gone well.
- One way to reduce overtreatment is to pay physicians a salary with a bonus for quality. When physicians are paid a salary, the number of tests and procedures decreases by 8–33 percent. Survey data show that doctors would support this shift to salary. The best care in the United States is provided by places that already pay by salary—some with no bonus—including the Mayo Clinic, Cleveland Clinic, and Kaiser Permanente. We should learn from them.

# Chapter Sixteen

# Myth: The United States Will Never Be Able to Reduce the Cost of Medical Care

## LET'S TALK "VALUE" BEFORE ATTACKING "COST"

We hear a lot of discussion in medicine about value. *Value* has a definition—quality divided by cost.[1] As discussed in chapter 6, it is difficult to get, for example, a health system to spend more money on medical care even if the actual value for the service is higher. Therefore we wonder if, in fact, the definition of *value* should be changed to "the improvement of outcome at the same or lower cost." For this chapter, as we consider how US health care could cut costs, we must be sure that quality stays the same or even increases. We must resist the idea that for a large decrease in cost, it is okay to let quality suffer a little.

## REDUCING THE COST OF MEDICAL CARE: START BY GETTING RID OF WASTE

To reduce waste, says Donald Berwick, former administrator of the Centers for Medicare and Medicaid services during the Obama administration, we must "keep processes, products, and services that actually help customers and systematically remove the elements of work that do not." Seems simple enough, right? "The challenge in removing waste from US health care," says Berwick, "will be to construct sound and respectful pathways of transition from business models addicted to doing more and more to ones that do only what really helps." These cost-saving measures also improve value—that is, they do not allow quality to suffer. Here we recall our discussion in chapter 3 (and table 3.1, specifically) and address each of the areas of waste Berwick identified.[2]

We begin our examination with waste created through administrative complexity.

## Administrative Complexity

### *Develop and Adopt Well-Functioning Electronic Health Records*

The most important way to reduce the waste due to administrative complexity is to have an electronic health record that is friendly to patients and physicians alike. Creating such software, obviously, is not so simple: about 90 percent of physicians use EHRs, whereas only 34 percent are satisfied with them.[3] While undoubtedly the user interface for patient records will continue to improve, at present many physicians struggle with operating the software and speaking with patients simultaneously, with the computer acting as both a real and a symbolic barrier between them. Many physicians hire scribes to put what the physician says into the record. Unfortunately, simply dictating doesn't work, given the way the records are structured. Solving this data-entry problem will allow doctors and health systems to harness the real power of EHRs to help them solve problems, as discussed below. A more friendly EHR is coming—just like the automobile replaced horses, and probably with almost as much angst.

### *Implement Decision Support through the Use of "Big Data"*

One other important part the EHR will play in cutting administrative waste is by providing *decision support*—in other words, helping health-care providers make the right call. In their current iteration, EHRs can perform relatively simple tasks, like searching for possible drug interactions based on medications a patient is currently taking. But imagine a true network of EHRs, where a patient's record could be accessed by any of their health-care providers, whether or not their providers are part of the same hospital or medical system. If the patient were to have a new problem, the record would know to "ask" certain relevant questions, based on the patient's history, to aid the physician in diagnosis. For example, the EHR would know that a patient has been prescribed aspirin by one doctor, so when the patient then goes to another doctor—who is unaware of this prescription—and describes stomach pain, the EHR would be "smart" enough to make the connection between the aspirin and stomach pain.

But this is "easy stuff." Artificial intelligence is improving, and IBM's Watson, for example, has already made some sophisticated diagnoses, properly identifying certain very rare conditions—as well as common conditions.[4] But for most patients, diagnosis isn't the real problem; the issue is how best to manage their condition. For starters, improved technology will one day be able to access and consider all medical literature across the entire globe before making recommendations. The EHR will have access to "big data," which will find a large number of patients with characteristics similar to those of the patient and exactly the same problem as the patient—as well as what different choices for management that were available and what happened. In the end, the EHR should "know" not only the patient but also the physician well enough to offer an array of treatment choices and eventually be "smart" enough to prioritize care options the same way the physician would. This type of technology won't be available next week, but it's the direction we're headed.

And now we turn our attention to another area of considerable waste in health care: the problem of overtreatment.

## Overtreatment

### *Eliminate Fee-for-Service Payment Models*

As we discussed in chapter 15, the bottom line is that if physicians were paid salaries—as opposed to being paid for every procedure or test they perform—medically unnecessary treatment would decrease, and the number of tests and procedures performed would fall by perhaps 20 percent, with about the same amount reflected in savings.[5]

### *Tie Payment to Guidelines*

Most physician groups—like the American College of Cardiology or the American Academy of Dermatology—provide practice guidelines to advise physicians on the best current treatments and practices. Some physicians adhere to the guidelines more than others. For example, 70 percent of cardiologists used guidelines frequently, compared to 47 percent of primary-care providers, 34 percent of other specialists, and 25 percent of orthopedic surgeons.[6]

To call attention to the problem, the American Board of Internal Medicine has initiated the Choosing Wisely campaign, inviting physicians create a list of procedures and tests that should *not* be performed in their area of medicine.[7] This is exactly the right approach to eliminating costs associated with unnecessary medical care.

## Use Practice Guidelines in Lawsuits

As guidelines are improving, they are more often used in lawsuits. If the guideline applies to a particular patient, the physician following the guideline can point to a guideline that has been "recommended" by their specialty physician organization. Guidelines can also be used to point out that the physician was not following the "standard of care." If a physician does something that the guidelines recommend they not do and a patient is hurt, the guidelines can help show error.[8] In the best case, the guidelines either agree or disagree with what the physician did and can be accepted as sufficient evidence, meaning that the expense of a trial could be avoided.

## Improve End-of-Life Care

The United States spends $205 billion annually on patients in their last year of life. This amounts to a staggering 13 percent of annual health-care spending.[9] Strategies around end-of-life care must focus on the patient's quality of life and on loved ones and provide as much information as possible. In a huge setback to better informing patients about their care options, former governor of Alaska Sarah Palin popularized the notion that the federal government planned to create "death panels" composed of government bureaucrats to determine which health services a person could receive or not receive at the end of life.[10] Palin's claims were completely false—there were no death panels and were never any plans for death panels—but the term and the resulting fear has remained. What the federal government *had* been discussing was finding ways to talk about the best end-of-life care options with patients and families—not curtail anyone's life. The most successful approaches to end-of-life care involve determining *advance directives*—or the recorded wishes of the individual patient and family. As the Mayo Clinic explains, "They guide choices for doctors and caregivers for patients that are terminally ill, seriously injured, in a coma, in the late stages of dementia or near the end of life."[11]

Advance directives provide written documentation of the patient's wishes: *Living wills* are written, legal instructions that explain what type of medical care a patient wants or doesn't want if the patient can't make decisions for themselves (e.g., "Do everything medically possible to keep me alive" or "Do not intubate me if I cannot breathe on my own"). The *medical* or *health-care power of attorney* is a person the patient empowers to make decisions for the patient when the patient is unable to do so. In some states this directive may also be called a *durable power of attorney for health care* or a *health-care proxy*.[12] The Mayo Clinic offers excellent considerations for choosing such a person.[13]

Advance planning for end-of-life care has the potential to improve quality of life as well as reduce expense. "Savings with significantly lower levels of Medicare spending occur with advance directives due to the lower likelihood of patients dying in the hospital and their more frequent use of hospice care."[14] Additionally, those who work to improve end-of-life care note that there often comes a point when more treatment doesn't necessarily equate to better care. A Dartmouth study, for example, examined the use of three life-sustaining treatments associated with end-of-life care: endotracheal intubation, feeding-tube placement, and CPR. These procedures can save lives, but in patients with advanced chronic illness, the chance that they'll prolong life is low. Even worse, these procedures can cause harm and prolong suffering. In some parts of the country, including Los Angeles and Chicago, more than 15 percent of patients receive these treatments during their last month of life. Yet patients who are more involved in their end-of-life care often decline to receive these treatments, which suggests that we're spending a lot of time, effort, and money administering interventions they don't actually want either.[15]

How do we address this problem? In 2011, a New York state law took effect that requires health-care providers to offer counseling regarding end-of-life and palliative care to patients expected to die within six months. New York officials say the law is not supposed to limit a patient's options but instead aims to permit patients to make choices that align with their own goals.[16] At one New York hospital, the percentage of terminal patients receiving palliative care tripled after the law took effect.

Unfortunately, having these conversations isn't the norm. For example, only 65 percent of nursing-home patients have an advance directive.[17] There is great opportunity to increase the frequency of these discussions, as studies have shown that up to 90 percent of nursing-home patients and families will complete advance directives if a physician initiates the discussion.[18]

*Empower Patients to Be Responsible*
*for Their Own Health and Health Care*

We would like to think that patients try to look up data about the quality of their physicians and the cost. But they don't. A Kaiser Family Foundation poll found that "only about 6 percent of people ever used quality information in making a decision regarding an insurer, hospital, or doctor. And fewer than 9 percent used information about prices. Only 3 percent of respondents said they used price information about physicians."[19]

Patients need better tools that speak to them at their level of education. Education is the key to helping people to make the best health and healthcare decisions. Insurers should encourage consumers to be good shoppers by making tools that rank cost and quality of care. Adding incentives by allowing patients to keep a portion of money they save when they are smart shoppers might be a way of encouraging them to make the right choice, since in many cases patients don't otherwise necessarily have any incentive to consider cost after reaching their deductible. It will be important that these tools balance cost and quality and not report only on cost.

By providing materials that patients can understand, there is a better chance that patients will actually follow doctors' orders and take responsibility for their own health. In order for *consumer-directed health care* to be effective, every consumer needs to be able to understand health information.

Remember that 40 percent of life expectancy is due to behavior and that risky behavior has a cost. If smoking and obesity were eliminated, US life expectancy would increase by about four years.[20] According to a 2017 survey conducted by the Texas Medical Center's Health Policy Institute, involving nine thousand consumers across fifteen states, consumers and physicians alike said individuals with bad health behaviors should pay more for health insurance.[21] The survey found that more than half of consumers endorsed a "fat tax" that involved charging more for food and drinks that could lead to obesity.[22] Three-quarters of respondents in the 2018 survey supported labels on menus and vending-machine items that indicate calorie counts or other information that signals whether a food is healthy.[23]

While incentivizing healthier choices could go a long way toward improving life expectancy—and cutting wasted health-care dollars—other behaviors including drug abuse, murders, and causing accidents must be addressed.[24]

*Improve Medication Adherence*

About half of patients with chronic diseases fail to take their medications appropriately, increasing their cost of care.[25] It saves us money when patients take their medicine as directed, even when considering the cost of the medicine itself, amounting to $7,900 per year for patients with heart failure and $3,900 per year for patients with diabetes.[26]

*Government Mandates*

We need to examine the effectiveness and cost of large government health programs. For example, home-health services are available to homebound people after hospital stays, with an annual program budget of $20 billion. The Centers for Medicare and Medicaid is taking a hard look at the value provided by these home-health services.[27]

What about state-mandated benefits for commercial insurance? Overall, there are 2,133 mandates across the fifty states—an average of forty-three per state. These mandates vary widely: for example, three states each mandate insurance payment for naturopaths, pastoral counseling, and athletic trainers, while eleven mandate hair prosthesis, but only thirty-four mandate diabetic self-management. In many cases, these mandates come as a specific request from one or more state legislators with little requirements for supporting data.[28] The country would do well to analyze these mandates and eliminate whatever isn't working.

While making these realistic changes to our system will undoubtedly reduce overtreatment, our health-care costs will still be far too high until we better target and eliminate fraud and abuse. And that is where we turn our attention next.

## Fraud and Abuse

Between 6 and 10 percent of all charges to Medicare and Medicaid are fraudulent.[29] For Medicare alone, this is $60 billion per year.[30] The most common type of Medicare fraud is committed by suppliers of durable medical equipment (things like walkers and wheelchairs), followed by physicians, hospitals, and home-health agencies.[31] In order for an act to be fraudulent and abusive, it must be intentional—that is, not accidental. At least a portion of fraud occurs because Medicare requires no preauthorization. A doctor, hospital, or home-care or medical-supply company sends a bill electronically, and a government check comes through the mail. When a physician bills Medicare for an hour to see a patient whom they really only spent about ten minutes with, this is fraud. If a physician bills for a patient they haven't seen at all that day, this, too, is fraud. Fraud can also be subtler, like requiring patients to return more frequently than necessary (for example, every other day) for a long period. Hospitals add "complications" to the charges, like billing for care of conditions like "fluid retention," which can occur in any-one and the reasonable treatment of which may not prolong length of the admission. Durable medical equipment suppliers may supply a cheaper wheelchair than they billed for.

Fraud and abuse occur not only in federal programs but also among commercial insurers. Much less fraud is committed in private insurance plans than in Medicare and Medicaid. Almost everything in commercial insurance requires preauthorization: expensive blood tests, scans, and procedures re-quire an explanation of the rationale and often require a phone call to a reviewing physician. Usually the policy of a private insurer is to not pay without preauthorization. The lesson from McAllen, Texas—while not an example of fraud—is important to remember: Media reports indicated that McAllen was the second-most expensive place to get medical care in the United States, based on Medicare payments per person.[32] But for commercial payers, it was at the median.[33] Why was this the case? Because Medicare permitted a lot that commercial insurers would not.

An early solution could be for the government to encourage private indus-try to produce automated-billing software that would be applicable for all physicians. The software reads the electronic health record and decides on the appropriate code, suggesting the code for the physician, and then carrying out the remainder of the process automatically. This type of automated bill-ing has been available for radiology for some time but could extend to all areas of medicine.[34] This process should reduce fraud, especially if the num-ber of times a code is changed to a more expensive one can be easily audited.

With better methods in place to reduce fraud, presumably some or many of the restrictions on EHRs standing in the way of efficient patient care can be eliminated.

## Pricing Failures

As discussed previously, the United States has higher prices for medical care than all other countries in the world. Among the numerous other reasons for this, Medicare is prohibited by law from considering how much something costs when deciding whether to pay for it. This prohibition extends back to the initial legislation that created the federal program.[35] Making matters worse, ACA makes it illegal for the federal government to use information on cost effectiveness in Medicare-coverage decisions. Currently, only *comparative-effectiveness* analysis is permitted. In other words, when determining which care should be provided, treatment effectiveness and potential for harm may be compared, but cost may not be considered. Imagine trying to buy a car without knowing the price.

Prescription drug costs in the United States illustrate this situation perfectly: According to a Commonwealth Fund report, per-capita drug spending on prescription drugs was higher in the United States than in all other nations. US prices are about three times those in the United Kingdom.[36] There are lessons to be learned from the United Kingdom on this topic: The National Institute for Health and Care Excellence is a nongovernmental body that provides essential health-care information, considers cost effectiveness in its analyses mainly of drugs, and creates practice guidelines. To develop these guidelines, NICE uses a formula that measures severity of disease, including both the quality and the quantity of life lived, measured in quality-adjusted life years (QALYs), as we discussed in chapter 3.[37] It's a model worthy of consideration, given the vast difference in drug costs between our two nations.

Changes to the FDA drug-approval process could help curb this waste. For example, increased speed of review for drugs that are potentially less expensive than existing drugs would possibly cause drug prices to fall.

Finally, Medicare has been prohibited from negotiating with drug companies on the price of prescription drugs. Plenty of people think that should change. The argument is unsettled. In 2007, the Congressional Budget Office determined that lifting the prohibition would not change prices much, as the government already does a lot of negotiating with drug companies—like, for example, the Veterans Administration.[38] However, it has been a long time since a thorough analysis of potential savings has been done. An up-to-date analysis would be worthwhile.

At a meeting in Houston with a number of health-policy luminaries, including two prior CMS administrators and a prior FDA commissioner, Garson asked each person, "Yes or no: the government must consider cost and cost effectiveness." Every one of the ten panelists responded with a resounding "yes."

## Failures of Care Delivery: Safety

Medical errors are truly a serious problem, and one might think that they should all be preventable. Most of the problems are associated with a few common events. The worst include health-care-associated infections, blood clots in the veins, pressure ulcers, medication error, and wrong or delayed diagnosis. It is estimated that every adult in the United States will experience an error in diagnosis at least once during their lifetime.[39] Many of these errors can be prevented—with the cost of preventing the error less than the cost of the negative effects of the error. For example, hospital-associated-infection- and blood-clot-prevention programs cost a fraction of the cost of the problems they cause. In cases where serious medical errors have been committed, usually a number of things have gone wrong at the same time. This is actually good, since prevention of just one of the problems might be able to prevent the entire error.

There has been great progress in prevention of medical errors. Aircraft pilots have taught us that checklists are important and effective: no matter how experienced the pilot, the takeoff checklist must be completed. And copilots have learned to question decisions made by the captain, preventing countless errors, which could be catastrophic. A similar top-down situation occurs in the operating room with the chief surgeon: the assistants learn that they must speak up if they notice potential problems. Every person in a hospital or clinic must think about these issues daily. And the care must extend beyond the professionals. It is well known that, when a hospital has problems with infections in the operating room, if every person at the facility—down to the janitors and technicians—begins carefully washing their hands, the problem usually disappears without identification of a single source.

Each of these changes can significantly improve our ability to keep patients safe and provide an excellent level of care. To further improve patient care, we must also address certain failures in care coordination that result in unnecessary hospital admissions and readmissions and that strain the resources of our emergency departments.

## Failures of Care Coordination

### Task Shifting

The United Kingdom has popularized *task shifting* in health care, which entails managing personnel so that expensive professionals are only performing tasks that they are uniquely capable of performing. Task shifting saves time and reduces costs by utilizing less expensive personnel to perform more routine tasks. Frequently, personnel lower in the organizational chain can actually perform the task more effectively, as they are interested in performing well when performing at the top of their capability. The top person in that case may feel the task is trivial. Task shifting means specialists primarily do work that only a specialist is suited to do, generalist physicians only perform work that physicians are suited to do, and so on and so forth, down the list. We don't want doctors doing work that nurse practitioners can do, for example, since nurse practitioners can do it at less cost and, in some cases, more effectively.[40]

If the United States aims to achieve health-care cost savings through task shifting, it must increase the use of nurse practitioners where appropriate and standardize curricula and certification for paraprofessionals as a pathway to public and private funding. Improving communication and task shifting has the opportunity to free up the primary-care physician to provide more specialty care and alleviate part of the specialty-care shortage.

Of course, the ultimate "task shift" is away from health-care professionals and to patients themselves. As discussed previously, when patients are empowered to make healthy, responsible choices—and given information in a manner that suits their needs—patients can avoid costly medical care. Just in the case of behavior, patients can save money by reducing overeating, smoking, and gun violence.

### Reduce Hospital Readmissions

Readmissions not only are costly but also interfere with the lives of patients and their families. Numerous attempts have been made to reduce readmissions. In a large study of six hospitals, researchers found that telephone calls from nurses and home monitoring of weight and blood pressure had no effect on readmissions.[41] The most effective strategy has been frequent home visits. Nurse practitioners making home visits were able to reduce readmissions for patients with heart failure by 48 percent, but the cost of the nurse practitioners was more than the cost of the readmission.[42] Grand-Aides—health-care assistants trained to assist in nursing care—reduced readmissions by 82 percent with net savings of more than $560,000 per year per Grand-Aide. [43]

*Reduce Emergency-Department Visits*

Emergency-department visits are expensive. A recent study discovered charges for treating strep throat at $328 in an ED, $130 at an urgent-care center, and $122 in a primary-care office. [44] The savings in avoiding ED visits and going to the proper level of medical facility could be more than $4 billion per year. [45] A significant number of ED visits are unnecessary, and many of these patients, in fact, could be managed at home. [46]

## THE BIG PICTURE

The cost of health care must be reduced significantly. We often hear talk of the need to "bend the cost curve"—meaning that it's acceptable to have prices increase, but the rate of increase just needs to slow down. [47] This is not good enough. As we have seen, we waste at least $1 trillion per year in the United States on health care. If we attack some of that waste successfully, we will decrease the cost of care, not just bend it. For example, in order to cover the uninsured, health insurance must be affordable—and that means decreasing the price of health care. If we are able to save by having less unnecessary tests and procedures ordered, the price of caring for a person will decrease. The best way to decrease the number of uninsured people is to make health insurance more affordable for everyone.

One of the most difficult problems in cost reduction in the health-care sphere is that someone's paycheck may rely on tests or procedures that are largely wasteful. This includes not just doctors but also nurses, technicians, administrators, and a whole slew of people associated with this line of work. For example, if we order fewer MRIs, some people—from MRI technicians to workers in the factories manufacturing imaging technology—will lose their jobs. With the shift away from inappropriate admissions and readmissions, fewer hospital beds will be needed. As hospitals close or downsize, people could be out of work. [48] In response to those pressures, MRI technicians should likely retrain for the next great diagnostic test, and hospital CEOs had better add more outpatient clinics.

In an ideal situation, everyone buys affordable health insurance and the first $200 billion of the wasted money will "fund" the insurance, meaning the money will still be in the health sector, paying insurance bills. But instead of that money paying for unnecessary health care for a smaller number of people, it will pay for necessary health care for a larger number of people. After that, there is every reason to think that taking the next $800 billion or so of waste out of the system will absolutely result in less money in the health sector. Investors, beware.

As painful as this is for some who make their living in the health sector—especially those in areas that are wasteful—in order for any meaningful health reforms to be instituted that increase coverage, the cost of health care must come down.

## CHAPTER SUMMARY

- To reduce the cost of medical care, we can attack the $1 trillion that we waste. Here are the big problems and possible solutions:

  - *Administrative complexity.* We need a well-functioning electronic health record system. Only a third of physicians find their EHR helpful. Ideally, the EHR gets to "know" patients and the type of support needed by the individual physician.
  - *Overtreatment.* We need to salary physicians to eliminate economic incentives that encourage them to overtreat, and we need to tie payment to practice guidelines published by physician associations.
  - *Fraud and abuse.* Between 6 and 10 percent of all charges billed to Medicare and Medicaid are fraudulent. Automated billing would reduce fraud and also free up more than one million billing clerks to learn a new trade.
  - *Pricing failures.* US prices for physicians, tests, and hospitalizations are higher than in the rest of the world. The United States has three times the cost of prescription drugs as the United Kingdom. The United Kingdom uses formal assessment of cost and years of life saved and only approves new drugs that have the best outcomes at the lowest cost.
  - *Failures of care delivery: safety.* Each year, medical errors kill more people than if a huge, full double-decker plane were to crash every day. Many of these medical errors can be prevented.
  - *Failures of care coordination: unnecessary hospital admissions and readmissions and emergency-department visits.* The best coordination is through teams, in which every member is working at the top of their skill level. For example, specialists should take care of the sickest pa-

tients, "task shifting" to generalists, and generalists should task shift to nurse practitioners.

- Looking at the big picture, as waste is decreased and the price of insurance decreases, more people will buy insurance. In order for any meaningful health reform to be enacted that increases coverage, the cost of health care must come down.

*Chapter Seventeen*

# Myth: When It Comes Right Down to It, Americans Are Like Everyone Else

When London hosted the Olympics in 2012, bright lights spelling out *NHS* shone from the stadium floor as a tribute to the National Health System that has served the British since the 1940s. The fact that the British showcased this system to the world shouldn't come as a surprise. In a recent poll, UK residents were asked to name what made them most proud to be British. Among the people who brought us Shakespeare, the royal family, and the BBC, more named the National Health Service than anything else. [1]

How confusing that was for Americans, who were so used to hearing about the dangers of "socialized medicine" during their political discourse at home. British director Danny Boyle explained why he included the NHS segment in the opening ceremony. "One of the reasons we put the NHS in the show is that everyone is aware of how important the NHS is to everybody in this country," he said at a press conference. "One of the core values of our society is that it doesn't matter who you are, you will get treated the same in terms of health care." [2]

Boyle is right that this is a key value of British society. But it is by no means a value of American society. We do not have a British-style health-care system because we are not British and we never will be.

Journalist T. R. Reid described our current health care well:

> In many ways, foreign health-care models are not really "foreign" to America, because our crazy-quilt health-care system uses elements of all of them. For Native Americans or veterans, we're Britain: the government provides health

care, funding it through general taxes, and patients get no bills. For people who get insurance through their jobs, we're Germany: premiums are split between workers and employers, and private-insurance plans pay private doctors and hospitals. For people over sixty-five, we're Canada: everyone pays premiums for an insurance plan run by the government, and the public plan pays private doctors and hospitals according to a set fee schedule. And for the tens of millions without insurance coverage, we're Burundi or Burma: in the world's poor nations, sick people pay out of pocket for medical care; those who can't stay sick or die.[3]

So who are we? It is important that we ask that question, because who we are as Americans and, indeed, how America works will ultimately determine the development of our eventual health-care system. We should plan for a true health-care system. What it looks like and when that occurs is the topic of the next few chapters.

In exploring who we are and how that affects our health-care system, we can best describe our American values through ten principles.[4]

## 1. RUGGED INDIVIDUALISM

The American rags-to-riches story is set in the national self-image of ideal-ism, opportunity, and sacrifice. The American dream perhaps first developed its sense of rugged independence in the Wild West and further defined its sense of dogged determination during the Depression years, in which one "pulled oneself up by the bootstraps," from poverty to wealth. The emphasis was on individual effort and responsibility in order to "make it." Many left grandchildren and great grandchildren quite wealthy with inheritances. Un-fortunately, some of the people who benefit from that system forget they didn't pull anything up by their *own* bootstraps, yet nonetheless feel that everyone else should be capable of achieving a rags-to-riches story.

In today's world, "making it" for a large number of people doesn't mean achieving wealth but simply finding a paying job. Those who insist that *Everyone can make it the way I (or my great-grandfather) did* might be surprised to know that about 85 percent of the uninsured come from working families, with 75 percent having a full-time job.[5] How can that be? The workers have to put bread on the table and a roof over their heads; yet many of them cannot not also afford health insurance, despite working as hard as they can. But the myth lives on that anyone can make it in America if only they try hard enough, and Americans hold a pervasive national attitude that looks at those who are struggling and says, *I'm not going to help you, because you shouldn't need my help.*

And how would this affect our health-care system?

Since American culture is rooted in the myth that everyone can make it, we are reluctant to provide our tax dollars to support someone else's health care. We are charitable as individuals. We will help our neighbors and will take a sick, uninsured coworker to the emergency department and might even pay for the visit. We perform amazing acts of kindness and humanitarian assistance in the face of natural disasters like Hurricane Katrina or Hurricane Harvey. But we have little interest in supporting large groups of "faceless" people, such as the unknown uninsured masses, over the long term. The I-can-do-it-myself philosophy is the basis for today's emphasis on consumer-directed health care, in which individuals are "empowered" to make decisions for themselves, without considering how those decisions might not always be the best even for them. We like what we call "freedom of choice" to choose—and keep—our own doctors. We are tolerant of multiple approaches to health care. But in the end, what we get is no "system" at all.

## 2. SIMPLE MESSAGE

Social media is very effective at priming us to receive certain messages. Most marketing communications are written to make it seem like the message is "speaking to me, directly," and the language is carefully chosen to give a short and simple personalized message. Often a fifteen-second video sound bite is all that is needed to get a viewer to buy into the message, and this subtle—and sometimes not-so-subtle—manipulation connects us, personally, to whatever the message represents.

And how would this affect our health-care system?

When it comes to complex medical information, Americans want something simple. For example, the concept of *quality medical care* is extremely complicated. Therefore, we prefer to choose our physician and hospital the same way we choose our auto mechanic: we take the recommendation of our neighbor, or we respond to effective advertising.

## 3. CONSUMERISM

Remember, we live in a country founded on the pursuit of happiness. This translates into a desire to have everything we want, and quickly—whether it's a fancy car, whitened teeth, or the latest pharmaceutical.

And how would this affect our health-care system?

We feel we have a right to whatever makes us happy and so, therefore, we have a right to health care—all that we want. Americans feel entitled to any available medical service, regardless of how much benefit it actually provides. We will not wait for a physician visit and will become angry if we do not receive a return phone call within minutes. Waiting lines? Absurd. Rationing? No way.

When it comes down to it, many Americans question whether we actually have a right to health care. There are a lot of definitions of *rights*, including whether something appears in the US Constitution. But entering into this conversation is not helpful, as we could spend hours debating the definition. Instead of insisting that Americans have a right to affordable health care, advocates should make the similar argument—and an argument that would cause fewer legal issues—that Americans should all have affordable health care.[6] Health care must be affordable not only to individuals but also to employers and society at large.

## 4. OPTIMISM

Patients and their loved ones are always "the exception" to any rule. For example, Joe is brought to the emergency department barely alive after an automobile accident. Yet even in the face of his grievous injuries, his wife rushes to his bedside, saying, "I know Joe will make it—he's always beaten the odds."

And how would this affect our health-care system?

Researchers have developed a system that can predict with 95 percent certainty whether an individual will leave an intensive-care unit alive.[7] It performed well in testing, but it was never accepted for use. Why? One reason that it failed was because, over and over, the patients' families were convinced that their relative was in the 5 percent who would live, all other evidence to the contrary. And this attitude is why we spend so much money in the last twelve months of a patient's life. In many Americans' minds, death is not an option.[8]

## 5. "IT'S THE ECONOMY, STUPID"

Our own personal finances as well as the economy of the country drive our views in so many areas. During the first presidential campaign of Bill Clinton, a sign hung in his campaign headquarters with campaign strategist James Carville's famous words, reminding staffers, "It's the economy, stupid."[9] Carville understood—and wanted everyone working to get Clinton elected to remember—that Americans go into the voting booth thinking mainly about their own personal finances. This is still true today.[10]

And how would this affect our health-care system?

In a good economy with high employment, fewer people are uninsured because more employers are able to offer insurance and workers have more money to purchase it. During those times, the issue of health-insurance coverage may disappear from the headlines. In a struggling economy, levels of unemployment and lack of insurance increase. As the economy continues to worsen, employers reduce the amount they are willing to pay for health insurance, either dropping coverage entirely or shifting more payment to the employee who is less able to pay the premiums. These actions increase the growing numbers of the uninsured.

## 6. THE THIRTY- TO FIFTY-YEAR LIBERAL-CONSERVATIVE CYCLE

In recent times, the attitudes of Americans have shifted every thirty to fifty years from conservative to liberal and back again. For conservatives, private companies rule, taxes are low, government is small, and individual responsibility is important; there is a deep belief in "traditional values." Then we switch to liberalism, which, in many ways, is the opposite philosophy: it looks to the government to protect the disadvantaged, usually through public programs paid for by taxing the "advantaged."

And how would this affect our health-care system?

It is clear from history that overall social and economic conditions have an important effect on how we feel about our health-care system at any given time. This reflects our willingness to tolerate the numbers of people living without insurance in this country. Our current view of health insurance favors continued involvement of the employer. We know we're in a conservative era when we come within one US senator's vote of taking health care away from twenty-three million people.[11] But this situation may be shifting.

There have been times in the past when America's views were more liberal, such as during the early 1960s, when two sweeping social programs were initiated: Medicare and Medicaid.

## 7. DIVERSITY OF OPINION

We are a country built on diversity of opinion. In political terms, we have "red" and "blue" states. Our elected officials must appeal to a wide variety of people of varying interests and priorities. Given this much diversity, agreeing on any large-scale national change is much less likely than taking small steps that offend the least number of people. Within each state, there is a bit more similarity among its citizens, bringing greater opportunities to advance more significant change that, at least, fits that particular state and its own views of diversity.

And how would this affect our health-care system?

With such diverse attitudes, we put up with many different types of systems. States that have populations more similar to one another—for example, Maine and Minnesota—are more likely to both take on initiatives that advance a particular goal, such as reducing the number of uninsured in the state. States are laboratories for change.[12] Many experts believe that letting states experiment with programs addressing health-care coverage and cost problems will be more feasible than large-scale efforts meant to apply to the entire country—at least in the short term.

## 8. MISTRUST OF GOVERNMENT

Any number of us have heard a neighbor say, *I don't need the government telling me what to do with my money. No more taxes.* Sound familiar? Our ethic of "rugged individualism" applies here as an attitude that is, by and large, antitax and antigovernment.

And how would this affect our health-care system?

With this mistrust of the government, many Americans do not want a "government-run" health-care system. They point their fingers at Canada's government-run program, with people waiting in line for treatment and traveling to Detroit for care. Americans criticize Canada's centralized system, even as they praise our own Medicare program, which, in many ways, looks very similar to Canada's system. We often read about seniors saying,

"I don't want a government system, but don't take my Medicare away!"—which doesn't make sense.

To most Americans, Medicare really isn't seen as a government program even though the government pays the bills, because Medicare offers free choice of physician, free choice of which hospital to go to, relatively short waiting times, and now even prescription drugs. In fact, Medicare may not even be seen as a government-paid system, since it's really like Social Security: seniors feel like they've paid into the system for years and are now getting what's rightfully theirs. For this reason, "Medicare for all" may be growing in popularity.

## 9. WE ARE INFLUENCED BY LOBBYISTS

Our politics are shaped to a real extent by lobbying—which is a way of life for much of Washington, D.C., and the state capitals. The largest industries spend millions of dollars on lobbying every year, and they're led by the health and medical sectors.[13] These groups are likely to influence policy for long into the future, because they provide generous campaign contributions for those running for office or, like the AARP, they represent large blocs of voters. Politicians ignore these influence peddlers at their peril.

And how would this affect our health-care system?

Pharmaceutical Research and Manufacturers of America, Blue Cross Blue Shield, the American Hospital Association, and the American Medical Association made political contributions totaling $20.4 million in 2018 alone.[14] Additionally, while not directly a health-care group, AARP certainly considers health care one of its major agenda items and is very influential with Congress because of the large voting bloc represented by senior citizens. But whichever group is doing the spending, lobbying is an effort to buy political influence. For example, as we have discussed previously, a major reason our government does not consider value to the patient when deciding what drugs are approved for use in the United States is that the pharmaceutical industry has effectively secured its own interests. Consideration of value could cause some drugs not to be approved and could decrease the cost of others in order to meet a cost-per-year-of-life-added benchmark.

## 10. WHAT THE FEDERAL GOVERNMENT AND
## STATES CONTROL IS VERY DIFFERENT

States are required to balance their budgets, whereas the federal government is not, which means that states are more limited in the financial investments they can make. However, states are natural laboratories of change because they can at times avoid the legislative gridlock at the federal-government level and thus be more innovative and responsive to their individual state needs. [15]

And how would this affect our health-care system?

The federal government has major power over taxation and therefore how much is paid for government health-care programs, since the federal government pays for all of Medicare and about half of Medicaid.

States regulate the licensing of doctors and medical malpractice. There are arguments for and against the need for different states to have different licensing and malpractice laws. Those in favor of state control largely use the argument that states are different, so different states should be allowed to govern themselves differently. Those who would rather see political power more centralized in the federal government, by contrast, point to the hassles, for example, of obtaining multiple state medical licenses in order to deliver telemedicine. States also determine many of the benefits within the Medicaid program, which has substantial variation from state to state based on income and because states may add their own requirements on to the basic federal requirements. Because states have different needs, state-based approaches to health care have been more popular nationally, generally in the form of getting waivers from the federal government to make changes in existing state programs.

## HOW AMERICAN VALUES INFLUENCE
## THE AMERICAN HEALTH-CARE SYSTEM

Lasting major health reform will have to reflect the underlying principles, values, and politics that make us who we are. This is not easy, partially because the interests are so varied and may be, at times, contradictory. For better or for worse—often, for worse—any US health-care-system reform will likely need to do the following:

1. Continue Medicare largely as is, as it works for those receiving, and those over sixty-five (the majority of whom receive Medicare) have the highest percentage of voters.[16]
2. Be consistent with desires of the lobbyists, including commercial insurance companies, drug and device companies, hospitals, doctors, and the AARP.
3. Provide patients a choice of physician and hospitals.
4. Require that patients spend little or no time waiting for services.
5. Don't ration health care.

These first five necessities for future health-care reform will likely have to be considered for a long time coming. But these next five may well change depending upon where we find ourselves in the liberal-conservative cycle:

1. Include no mandates.
2. Continue employer-sponsored health care.
3. Do not create a tax-supported, government-run system.
4. Keep Medicaid essentially intact.
5. Provide health care for everyone.

Not only will these considerations be required in any future health-care reform before Americans are satisfied, but the sun, moon, and stars in the liberal-conservative cycle must also be aligned. Does this mean that change in the American health-care system is impossible? We will explore this question in future chapters.

## CHAPTER SUMMARY

- Americans aren't just like everyone else. We don't have a British health-care system because we are not British.
- Our unique characteristics include our rugged individualism, our optimism, and our mistrust of government.
- Any approach to US health-care-system reform in the foreseeable future will likely need to do the following to be politically feasible:

  - Continue Medicare as is.
  - Be consistent with desires of the lobbyists including commercial insurance companies, drug and device companies, hospitals, doctors, and the AARP.

- Provide choice of physician and hospital to consumers.
- Require that there be little or no waiting for services.
- Avoid rationing of health care.

## Chapter Eighteen

# Myth: Previous Attempts at Health-Care Reform Have Taught Us Very Little

The George Santayana quote is a cliché because it's true: "Those who cannot remember the past are condemned to repeat it."[1] As we study the health-care system and ways to reform it, it's critically important that we remember we've had these debates before. Rather than bury them as ancient history, we must study these previous efforts and draw on them as we constantly strive to design better policy.

We can learn from every previous attempt at health reform. And we have plenty of source material to draw on, since every president since Franklin D. Roosevelt has dealt with national health care.[2] However, this book isn't meant to be an all-encompassing history, so let's begin with lessons from Bill and Hillary Clinton's efforts in the 1990s. At the end of the chapter, we'll offer insights into how we can apply lessons from that experience and others as we consider future efforts at health reform.

THE CLINTONS AND THE HEALTH SECURITY ACT: 1992–1994

To develop and monitor plans to overhaul the US health-care system, First Lady Hillary Rodham Clinton convened a task force of five hundred.[3] As the *New York Times* reported, "The staff was bigger than 99 percent of all businesses in the United States."[4] Here is what the proposed Clinton plan offered:

- All Americans had coverage. There was an individual mandate.
- Subsidies were given to low income people to help buy insurance.
- Standard benefits were required of all plans, including medical treatment and prescription drugs. There was no preexisting-condition exclusion.
- "Managed competition" was meant to manage health plans and insurers. Prices were set, including payment to physicians. There were caps on spending.[5]
- The health maintenance organization (HMO) was put forward as a delivery model. Under an HMO, doctors, hospitals, clinics, and an insurance company would all be working together. Primary-care physicians became gatekeepers to specialized care, meaning the only way a patient could see a specialist was with a referral from the PCP. Only certain doctors could be in a specific HMO.
- All employers were to either contribute to insurance for their employees or provide it (employer mandate) with government subsidies for small business to help them pay for insurance. Employers with more than five thousand employees could opt out and form their own plan as long as it met certain criteria.
- A National Health Board would set a health budget for the nation. It was to regulate most private health-insurance premiums and set national guidelines for determining which treatments could be provided and how often approved treatments or tests could be performed.
- Savings were planned through cost controls, greater efficiency, and preventive care as well as cutting Medicare and Medicaid spending. The only tax increase proposed for individuals was an additional cigarette tax. However, if the overall savings to pay for the plan were not achieved, individuals would pay higher taxes to make up the difference.

The original act was 1,342 pages long; it was never voted on and died in the latter part of 1994.

What did we learn?

1. The reaction to the Clinton plan was overwhelmingly negative. There are several reasons for this result. For starters, the potential for marked tax increases for individuals was not popular. The American dream, for better or for worse, does not involve higher taxes to take care of your uninsured neighbors. Additionally, both the individual and the employer mandates proposed in the plan were unpopular. And few

people—especially physicians and hospitals—wanted a government board deciding how frequently tests should be done. The plan's architects likely underestimated how much Americans valued the ability to choose their own doctors.

2. Then-Senator Robert Dole, a Republican representing Kansas, summed up the national feeling: "Turning over one-seventh of our economy to the United States government is an idea that has many Americans—Republicans and Democrats—very concerned."[6] We learned—once again—that the American people do not take to major change well, and this plan was as major as could be, in that virtually everything in the health system was poised to change.

3. Initially, the Clinton plan sought to insure the thirty-six million people in the United States who were then lacking health insurance. But critics highlighted the fact that those who *did* have insurance tended to be happy with the existing system and wouldn't take kindly to change. "Approximately 86 percent of Americans are covered by health insurance. Polls show they are overwhelmingly satisfied," the conservative Heritage Foundation wrote at the time.[7] We learned that to attack something that 86 percent of Americans had and to propose replacing it with an unproven system would not wash with the American people.

4. On a more superficial level, critics complained that the bill was long and complicated and that Hillary Clinton chaired the committee. This was like reading the title of a proposal, deciding you don't like it even before reading through it, and then looking for reasons to justify your dislike. Did it really matter how long the bill was or who was chairing the committee? Not really. But it was easier to complain about that than arguing the technicalities of changing an entire health system. Attitudes about the bill were completely along party lines, but even Democrats put forward a number of competing proposals.

## BARACK OBAMA AND THE AFFORDABLE CARE ACT: 2010 TO PRESENT

After Barack Obama's election to the American presidency in 2008, he and his Democratic allies in Congress quickly began working on what would become the signature policy achievement of his administration. "Obamacare," as this plan to reform US health care came to be known, was neither expected nor intended to achieve universal coverage but meant to expand insurance to more people. Obama signed the ACA into law in March 2010, just over a year after taking office. What did it do?[8]

- By calendar year 2019, the number of uninsured was projected to be reduced from fifty-seven million to an estimated twenty-three million.[9]
- Coverage would increase for the uninsured by expanding Medicaid eligibility from the lowest-income people up to those earning 138 percent of the federal poverty level ($16,753 for an individual in 2018[10]).

  - However, the ACA hit a snag: the US Supreme Court ruled that the Medicaid expansion would be optional.
  - As of April 2019, thirty-seven states, including Washington, D.C., have expanded Medicaid.

- For those individuals and families with incomes above 138 percent of the poverty level ($16,753) but below 400 percent ($48,559), states would have a state-based "marketplace exchange" mechanism, similar to the one in place in Massachusetts, where individuals shop for insurance coverage. The exchanges also managed subsidies for those who fell into this income range. However, we learned that the subsidies were inadequate for many low-income Americans.
- There were several parts to insurance reform. The most important were as follows:

  - The preexisting-condition exclusion was eliminated, meaning insurers could no longer deny coverage for people who had been diagnosed or treated for any condition the insurer decided to exclude.
  - Children up to age twenty-six could be covered by their parents' insurance program.
  - There were no lifetime limits for insurance payments for an individual or family.
  - There was an individual mandate that everyone have insurance or pay a penalty. This was unpopular, as it was seen as a penalty on those who didn't have the resources to buy insurance. It was repealed in 2017.
  - There were mandates for both small employers (fifty to two hundred employees) and large employers (more than two hundred employees) to provide health insurance to their employees.
  - All plans were required to have ten essential benefits: "ambulatory patient services (outpatient services), emergency services, hospitaliza-

tion, maternity and newborn care, mental-health and substance-use-disorder services, including behavioral-health treatment, prescription drugs, rehabilitative services (those that help patients acquire, maintain, or improve skills necessary for daily functioning) and devices, laboratory services, preventive and wellness services and chronic-disease management, [and] pediatric services, including oral and vision care."[11]

- Insurance rates for young, healthy people increased after the ACA took effect, because it established a maximum difference in insurance costs between eighteen-year-olds and sixty-four-year-olds at 300 percent. Since the rate for the older people needed to be as high as possible, this had the effect of increasing the rate for the younger people, too.
- Medicare coverage for prescription drugs increased.[12]
- $10 billion were earmarked to fund the new Center for Medicare and Medicaid Innovation, a laboratory for cost and quality. It was to stimulate value-based funding including accountable-care organizations, bundling, and capitation.
- Importantly, despite all of these reforms, the ACA did little to directly address issues of health-care costs or quality.

What did we learn?

1. At the time of the ACA debates, attitudes about the bill fell squarely along party lines. Favorable attitudes came from Democrats. The law, nicknamed "Obamacare," became personal, representing all things that Republicans disliked about the Democratic president. The demonization of Obamacare continued into the Trump administration, with the new president shedding anything he could that the Obama administration had done, leading the efforts to "repeal and replace" the law.
2. Because the ACA made no attempts to decrease the cost of care, the price of insurance kept increasing, making insurance unaffordable even for those with subsidies. For many individuals making $30,000 to $40,000, subsidies were insufficient to cover premiums and deductibles. Of course, affordability was even more challenging for those who didn't get subsidies at all.
3. The theoretical "insurance spiral" did occur. The concept describes the rising rates the people who continue to have insurance have to pay as more and more healthy people exit the insurance pools. The purpose of a preexisting-condition exclusion—as awful as the idea is—was to

stimulate healthy people to buy insurance. The idea was that the healthy would be worried that an accident or new, expensive disease could befall them in the future, causing them to buy insurance now. Without the preexisting-condition exclusion and with a weak individual mandate that was ultimately repealed, there was not any stimulus for some healthy people to buy health insurance, leaving sick people with higher and higher rates—hence the "the insurance spiral."

4. Remember President Obama's promise that everyone would be able to keep their own insurance after the ACA went into effect? Before the ACA, more than three million people had plans with high charges and skimpy benefits. The ACA declared these plans illegal, as all plans going forward would have to have the "ten essential benefits" referenced above. Those who had the plans became furious that they could not keep them—likely because they didn't really know what their plan consisted of and had never tried to use it but were nonetheless upset that what they had was being taken away. Though some may have been upset that they ultimately had to give up their plans, it's likely many of these people would have been even more upset had they ever actually tried to use their insurance, only to discover that their "coverage," in fact, covered very little, leaving huge bills for them to pay.

5. The US Supreme Court also limited aspects of the ACA that might have made the law more effective. The original law contained a clause stating that if a state failed to expand Medicaid to all people up to 138 percent of the poverty level, all the state's Medicaid payments from the federal government would be discontinued. The court held that this clause was too "coercive"—meaning that there was too great a penalty for not agreeing to do what the government wanted. The court made Medicaid expansion voluntary for each state. This initial crack in the dam widened as many saw that parts of the ACA could be made voluntary or repealed, and legal challenges to the law continued. In 2019, twenty state attorneys general brought a lawsuit to declare the ACA unconstitutional. If they win, the United States will go back to 2008, but with much more expensive health care.

6. Perhaps most important, we learned that a bill that passes into law with no support from the other party will last just as long as it takes to get a majority of the opposing party in Congress. For this reason, future attempts at major change must involve both parties from the very beginning.

## DONALD TRUMP AND THE AMERICAN
## HEALTH CARE ACT: 2017

The AHCA was presented as the way to repeal and replace Obamacare, a longtime campaign promise of Trump and many Republicans. What did it do?[13]

- All mandates—individual and employer—from Obamacare were repealed.
- Medicaid funding was changed entirely to become a *per-capita cap*, which provided a certain amount per person—and was therefore sensitive to changes in the number of covered people. But no one had any real idea whether the amount of the "cap" would come close to paying the actual expenses of the people. This became the mechanism for the federal government to severely reduce Medicaid funding. The cap was "sold" to state governors, who were told that they would have much more control over their state's money; the part the sellers didn't really mention was that the amount of money the governors would control would be a whole lot less.
- All funding for Medicaid expansion through the Affordable Care Act was discontinued, leaving fourteen million who had previously had Medicaid uninsured. Medicaid cuts totaled $880 billion over ten years.[14]
- Overall, AHCA would take insurance away from twenty-three million people previously covered through Obamacare—including those on Medicaid—resulting in fifty-one million uninsured by 2026, the greatest number of uninsured since before Medicare and Medicaid were introduced.[15]
- The maximum difference in insurance rates was changed so that younger people would have a rate that was 20 percent of the rate for older people (rather than 33 percent under ACA), thus lowering rates for young people.
- To incentivize people to buy insurance and keep it, insurers would increase the price of insurance by 30 percent for those who went without coverage for two months.
- States were permitted to repeal the ten essential benefits of the ACA.
- States could charge higher rates for people with preexisting conditions as long as they had a high-risk pool. They could still say they were providing coverage for preexisting conditions, even if the price was not affordable.
- Taxes on the wealthy were cut by $300 billion over ten years.

- The original savings were calculated to be $324 billion; eventually, the estimate was revised down to $150 billion, with little discussion.
- The bill passed the US House of Representatives, with all Republicans and no Democrats voting in its favor. The bill required fifty-one votes in the Senate to move forward, but it failed when three Republican senators voted against it. Had Senator John McCain voted for the bill, it would have passed and become law.

What did we learn?

1. The wave in the House of Representatives to approve the American Health Care Act was so strong that almost anything would have passed with a very strong president—at that time—and a majority of Republicans in the House and Senate. A few Republicans in the Senate who broke with their party ultimately killed the legislation. This is an important lesson for the future and a way to get major change enacted. The president and virtually all Republican lawmakers came within one vote of taking health insurance away from twenty-three million people with little concern, as if they were just a line on a piece of paper to be x-ed out.

2. Campaign promises, usually forgotten, were not forgotten in this case. Trump was elected and decided that his campaign promise to repeal Obamacare was a mandate when it was not. He then carried repeal and replace over to Congress, where members were forced to vote on the campaign promise with little to no debate, since voting against it would be disloyal. Trump delivered what many congressional Republicans had long campaigned on. After years of frequent votes in the House to repeal Obamacare, the GOP was suddenly the dog who caught the car. Ultimately, division within the party just barely prevented the GOP from repealing the law it had argued against for years. But it could have easily gone the other way.

3. The repeal of Obamacare became so important to the GOP that some provisions were not fully debated. For example, the amount of the subsidies relating only to age and not to income did not make sense. The reduction in the savings from $340 billion to $150 billion—meaning, therefore, the new bill would have a much smaller impact on reducing the deficit—received no public discussion.

4. The change in Medicaid funding to a per-capita cap was the means by which Medicaid funding would be reduced. State governors were on board with the plan when they were told it would give them "more control of funds."[16] This sounded great to the governors. What most did not realize was that, had the bill passed, they would have had control over a much *smaller* budget. Again, this facet of the bill was one of a tide of campaign promises that extended to the states. Critics of the provision argued that the reduction in Medicaid was a way to pay for the $300 billion tax cut on the wealthy.[17]

5. As many ACA provisions as possible were changed. Annual and life-time caps eliminated by the ACA were brought back in the new bill. No-cost preventive care was repealed, along with the requirement for the ten essential benefits. However, young people would still be able to remain on their parents' insurance, and the preexisting-condition exclusion remained.

The bill never became law, though it came awfully close. In the aftermath we have learned that campaign promises by any candidate must be taken seriously, and, therefore, major debate should occur around them. Candidates must be pressed to present real plans subject to real debate.

## SHORT- TO MEDIUM-TERM FIXES BASED ON WHAT WE HAVE LEARNED

How do we use these lessons to help us fix US health care? We'll cover longer-term plans for health reform in the next two chapters. But here are some reforms that can be either singly or together—independent of a massive health-care overhaul—employed to improve our system in the short term.

1. We must reduce the price of health care significantly and watch quality carefully to be certain value does not decrease even as we bring costs down. This can be done without any other action and should be done immediately. The first act should be to permit Medicare to consider cost and cost effectiveness in what it pays for. Lowering costs would make any attempts to cover more Americans with health insurance much more affordable. Lower health-care costs would also make it easier for small businesses to provide health insurance to their employees, with fewer people remaining uninsured or on Medicaid.

Medicaid dollars would stretch further, with lower costs, perhaps extending the safety net to more people. Finally, reduced costs could slow the death spiral of insurance. We have found in our Texas Medical Center surveys that 98 percent of Americans want insurance; the problem is that some just can't afford it. [18]

2. Value-based care (paying for quality) should be stimulated by offering incentives for value-based payment through capitation or bundling. It can also be stimulated via value-based payment to current hospitals and by paying physicians a salary with a bonus for quality, rather than reimbursing physicians through traditional fee-for-service payment models.

3. Insurance companies should get together as soon as possible and create insurance products that people can afford. These products would be for the individual or small-group market—and should provide only catastrophic care. They should be affordable, meaning they must have a low deductible, and they'd need to be something that large numbers of people would buy. Importantly, these types of plans can't simply be inexpensive, because they cover virtually nothing, as we've seen in the past.

4. We should develop a system to provide an incentive to consumers in order to encourage them to maintain continuous health-insurance coverage. [19] For example, those who maintain coverage would receive a credit toward a health-savings account. Such a step would need to be carefully analyzed to determine how great the overall savings might be were more healthy people to buy insurance.

5. We must work toward improving electronic health records so that they can be a real help to physicians and hospitals. Currently the EHR systems are seen by physicians as requiring more time with little benefit. These records should soon be able to bring improved decision support to physicians, improving care at lower cost. The government could stimulate innovation in automated billing for all services, reducing the likelihood of fraud and reducing billing expense.

6. The health-care safety net could be strengthened by increasing the number of federally qualified health centers. In addition to increasing the number, the FQHC program should pay for specialists and hospitalization, which it currently (basically) does not. The program should be upgraded to help deal with the increasing numbers of uninsured.

7. Much of what was learned in previous attempts at reform will be helpful as plans are made for the next major effort to change how coverage is delivered so as to cover all Americans with adequate health care. The major learning from the recent attempt and near success of the AHCA is that a single candidate with a campaign promise that lit a fire under his party was able to produce legislation that would have seriously hurt millions of people into the future. Popular enthusiasm for important policy decisions, properly directed, and absolutely with bipartisan support from the beginning, is the way to move forward for the benefit of all Americans.

8. We should begin health-care reform with state demonstrations. States could apply for federal grants for infrastructure to support experimentation in health-care reform. The Health Partnership Act legislation that Garson helped develop showed how that could be done by positing states as laboratories of health-policy innovation.[20] Each year, the states participating in the health-policy experimentation would convene to see what mutual learning has occurred with an eye to eventually taking the best practices and applying them nationally.

## CHAPTER SUMMARY

- Hillary Clinton's health-care plan in the 1990s taught us that

  - Americans reject tax increases—especially individual tax increases—even to help others. Their goal isn't to spend more to help the uninsured.
  - Americans care a lot about their ability to choose their own physician.
  - "Turning over one-seventh of our economy to the government has many Americans very concerned," as Senator Dole put it.

- We learned important things from the passage of the Affordable Care Act, too:

  - The legislation didn't address cost, so—no surprise—the price of insurance kept increasing, making insurance unaffordable even for those with subsidies. We learned that any future attempt at reform must start with cost reduction.

- Making Medicaid expansion optional eventually doomed the law and inspired legislators to try to repeal other parts of the law.
- Having a law as a signature of one party and president made it a personal target for the next administration. Future attempts at reform must be bipartisan.

- In 2017, Trump and the GOP provided lessons as well:

  - Campaign promises, usually forgotten, were not forgotten this time around. Trump carried his promise to "repeal and replace" Obamacare all the way to Congress, which was forced to vote on it. We learned to take campaign promises seriously and that major debate, therefore, should occur around them.
  - The wave in the House of Representatives to approve the American Health Care Act was so strong that almost anything would have passed. In the future, such a wave with a strong president and aligned Congress could enact major change.
  - It appeared that lawmakers would have passed nearly anything that was against Obama—and Obamacare was a prime target—and came within a vote of dramatically increasing the number of uninsured to the largest number the United States would have seen since before Medicare and Medicaid were established, all in service of the goal to "kill anything Obama."

## Chapter Nineteen

# Myth: Americans Are So Divided That We Can't Even Agree on Goals for Our Health Care

In 2000, when he was president of the American College of Cardiology, Garson proposed goals for the US health-care system: universal coverage, public and private payers, alternative to employer-based health insurance, administrative simplification, access to the right provider at the right time, improved health-care quality, new expense for the uninsured paid by redirecting current revenue, new revenue, and increased efficiency.[1] Sound familiar? These are virtually the same goals that conservatives and liberals have proposed in their various plans to reform our health-care system; yet somehow we continue to fail to make meaningful, lasting reforms. We express the goals in this chapter by focusing on the three targets that comprise US health care: the people, the practitioners, and the system itself. The issue that has plagued America is how to achieve those goals. We deal with that topic in chapter 20.

GOAL 1—FOR THE PEOPLE: COVERAGE FOR ALL WITH
ACCESSIBLE, AFFORDABLE, ADEQUATE HEALTH CARE

### Coverage

In the past, the term *universal coverage* was equated with single payer or "socialized medicine." Fortunately, these inappropriate definitions have been used less frequently of late; "coverage for all" seems to provide a clearer picture. How do we obtain 100 percent coverage for all Americans? The best approach in the relatively short run is to reduce the price of health care so that more people can afford the premiums and deductibles. For those who still fall through the cracks, funding could be increased to federally qualified health centers (FQHCs) that could then increase access to specialists and hospitals.[2] This increase could be jointly funded by the federal government—as it is now—as well as by states and counties.

The only way to eventually attain this goal is to create a "single safety net" for all people. (We discuss this in detail in chapter 20.) The rest sounds simple enough, but "accessible, affordable, adequate health care" means different things to different people. To optimists, it means "everyone has health insurance." For pessimists, it means everyone who can pay for insurance gets health care.

## Accessible

The appropriate use of the term *access* in health care means that a person can see the right medical practitioner for their needs, at the right time, and in the right place. For the insured, that may mean a typical doctor's office. But access can also mean care is available at a safety-net clinic or hospital—such as an FQHC or county hospital. The "right place" is an evolving concept. Today it might even mean a consult via e-mail or video call. But the right place does not mean the emergency department when we're talking about conditions like colds and sore throats.

How does everyone get access to care? One of the best ways is to have health insurance. But insurance alone is not sufficient. Talk to the people in rural America, or even urban people who are homebound and find it extremely difficult to get to a physician. They have health-insurance coverage, but there are few or no practitioners near them. It is worth underlining this difference: 100 percent access with 0 percent coverage means obtaining health care in the emergency room, as all people have access to a practitioner; 100 percent coverage and little or no access is what many Americans face in certain rural parts of our country. For example, once a year, for two days, there's a "clinic" that's set up in a huge parking lot in southwest Virginia where physicians and dentists provide free care. Since 1985, there have been volunteers at the clinic who have helped to care for about 750,000 people. The line to get in stretches over half a mile.[3] "The patient parking lot will open no later than midnight," the event organizer writes on its website.

"Numbered patient admission tickets will be given out beginning at 3 A.M., one ticket per patient. Clinic doors will open at 6 A.M. Patients will be admitted in numerical order by ticket number, and a ticket is required for admission."[4] This is one way we deliver medical care in the country. At least these people have *some* care.

For people in rural America, the best access to care they might have may mean an improved telemedicine program to connect doctors or nurses virtually with the patient, as well as a system of telemedicine support with specialists and perhaps other generalists for the few rural physicians or nurse practitioners.

As we have seen, nurse practitioners (NPs) are more likely to practice in rural areas than physicians.[5] The National Academy of Medicine recommended that NPs be permitted to prescribe all drugs and practice independently of a physician.[6] As of 2017, twenty-four states granted this independence to NPs.[7] However, the other states require physician oversight wherever NPs practice, usually due to strong lobbying by physicians.[8] Those states with restrictions have fewer rural NPs than those without restrictions.[9] By definition, areas where NPs would be providing the only access to care have no physicians, and therefore no physicians are available to provide oversight. At present, NPs are less expensive than physicians. Part of the reason is that most public and private payers only pay NPs 80–85 percent of the amount paid to physicians for the same service. Hopefully the difference in payment rate will be abolished. At present, even allowing for the difference in payment rates, NPs are still 17–24 percent less expensive than physicians due to reduced ordering of tests and procedures.[10]

"Young people who grew up in rural areas are four times more likely to practice [medicine] in places like the ones in which they grew up."[11] Medical school admissions policy could include more focused recruitment of students who grew up in rural areas and who say they are committed to returning to a rural practice; additional ways to increase physician numbers in rural areas include paying rural practitioners more money, locating medical schools in rural areas, and exposing physicians and nurses to rural health early in their education.[12]

FQHCs or community health centers provide access to the uninsured. More than half of these clinics are in rural areas.[13] As important as the care provided by FQHCs is, for some patients access to care may be limited, as some FQHCs do not have agreements with specialists or hospitals, mostly due to the FHQC's inability to afford the payments.[14]

## Affordable

What exactly does *affordable* mean? Thanks to new survey data, we actually have a precise answer. The Texas Medical Center's Health Policy Institute worked with a national firm to survey more than nine thousand individuals across fifteen states to gauge their views of the health-care system.[15] The section below explains what they told us about affordable health care.[16] More than 98 percent of respondents said they want insurance for themselves and their family. The so-called "invincibles" in their twenties and thirties who say they don't need health insurance are few and far between. Virtually everybody wants and sees the value of health insurance.

The problem, of course, is that many of them can't afford health insurance. That's not a surprise. When the drafters of the Affordable Care Act wrote the law in 2010, they emphasized "inexpensive" premiums. Well, the premiums were affordable for some (and fewer as the years went on), but the law did not focus on the deductibles—the amount consumers have to spend before their insurance really kicks in—for all but the lowest-income people. Those deductibles, well over $6,000 for some plans offered on the ACA exchanges, when combined with high premiums are why insurance is seen by the public as unaffordable.

We asked people in the survey who did not have health insurance what percentage of their income they considered an affordable amount to spend on health-care expenses, including the premiums and deductibles they pay as well as other out-of-pocket expenses, such as drug co-pays.

Well over half of the uninsured respondents said that 2–5 percent of income was an affordable amount to spend on health care; that included 60 percent of those earning at least $75,000 per year. We also saw similar results for respondents who had health insurance.

Cynics have argued that if people would only give up their luxury items—the latest smartphones, fancy televisions, luxury cars—they could afford to spend more on health care. Our survey data show that's not the case. Half of our respondents, whether they were insured or not, said they had to make significant cuts just to pay for health care. Across all incomes, they cut back in three areas to pay for health care: savings, clothing, and food. It's a troubling trend, given that most Americans have less than $1,000 in their savings accounts. For them, health care isn't just a health issue—it's an economic issue.[17]

But under the present law, coverage is considered affordable only if the premium doesn't cost more than 8.2 percent of one's income, compared to the 2 percent that survey respondents told us was actually affordable.[18] Therefore the government's "affordable" is four times the amount that citizens say is affordable. Consumers and lawmakers aren't speaking the same language when they talk about affordable health care. In the future, legislators need to understand what their constituents consider to be affordable so that they are not writing bills expecting people to buy insurance when they are not able to pay for it.

## Adequate

When we talk about *adequate* care, we're talking about the care that everyone needs. Admittedly, *need* is challenging to define. We alluded to this issue we discussed rationing. We believe that sooner rather than later discussions on what basic level of service everyone needs must take place. It is likely, given current prices, that we probably cannot even afford basic health care for all.[19] Of course, basic health care meeting mere *need* is less than the care that everyone might *want* to have.

## GOAL 2—FOR PRACTITIONERS: PAY BASED ON QUALITY, AND ELIMINATE HASSLES

According to Donald Berwick, past administrator of the Centers for Medicare and Medicaid Services, every year health-care providers waste $192 billion on *overtreatment*—or medically unnecessary care.[20] For example, in West Virginia heart procedures are performed at seven times the rate they're performed in San Francisco, even though West Virginians aren't seven times as sick. From this we take that many in West Virginia did not need the procedure and were overtreated. There are a number of possible reasons for this overtreatment, but an important one is that the doctors doing these procedures are paid for each one under a fee-for-service payment scheme. In the majority of cases, the doctor does not consciously overtreat the patient, but, whatever the reason for the unnecessary care, when physicians move from fee-for-service to salary, the number of procedures and tests done drops between 9 and 33 percent.[21]

The largest payer in the United States—the one that covers Medicare and Medicaid—has recognized overtreatment and has committed to paying physicians at least 50 percent using a value-based payment. This would not be a fee-for-service payment that reimburses for quantity; instead, value-based payment is based on quality. The most sensible way to deliver value-based care is to pay physicians a salary. There's precedent for this. In the highest-quality health-care systems in the nation, including the Mayo Clinic, Cleveland Clinic, and Kaiser Permanente, physicians are paid salaries—in most cases with a bonus based on quality. The salary could be at the same level the physician is making now, or slightly less with a real bonus added to make the total higher. The bonus could be based on patient satisfaction or on outcomes such as reducing readmissions to the hospital, among many others. Some payers worry that when physicians are paid a salary, they will see fewer patients (i.e., not work as hard); this is why we propose a quality bonus that does include, for example, a minimum number of patients seen and a patient-satisfaction metric saying "My practitioner spent enough time with me." Interestingly, physicians agree with us. In a recent survey conducted by the Texas Medical Center's Health Policy Institute, we found that 69 percent of doctors indicated their preferred method of payment was a salary.[22] Paying physicians salaries could save at least 10–15 percent of the total expense of health care since the incentive to do more to be paid more would decrease.[23]

What needs to happen for value-based care to work—meaning care would cost less but create the same or even better outcomes? Several things: First, these savings must be passed along to the consumer in the form of lower costs for their health insurance so that it becomes affordable. Second, commercial payers (big health-insurance companies) as well as the public payers (Medicare and Medicaid) should require that physicians be paid by salary. For single physicians and small groups, this might not actually be possible. For them, the payers should develop other incentives to reduce unnecessary tests and procedures. Why does this matter to patients? The number of unnecessary tests and procedures will decrease. Patients will not be exposed to the risks of these procedures. With more time available, physicians will hopefully be able to spend more time with patients, and, in the best of all worlds, the eight-minute doctor visit will be replaced by longer visits—more satisfying to both doctors and patients.

The second part of this goal for practitioners is that care should be hassle-free, including the use of well-functioning electronic health records (EHRs). Unfortunately, EHR systems have had an extremely rocky beginning, with large numbers of physicians claiming they're expensive to both buy and operate, as the poor design caused doctors to spend a lot more time fussing with the software, causing a real decrease in the numbers of patients they could see.[24] Physicians now spend only 55 percent of their working time in direct care of patients, with the rest spent dealing with the EHR and adminis-trative tasks.[25] Additionally, think about this: the government strongly stimu-lated physicians and hospitals to buy and use EHRs, and many did. And the companies producing many of them failed—causing another round of physi-cians spending money to buy new EHRs. Small physician practices could not afford such losses. It seems appropriate for the federal government to inject funding into practices who lost money while trying to meet federal require-ments. It has been said that the technology is currently available that would create a well-functioning, hassle-free EHR, but funds for the dissemination and infrastructure are needed. It seems appropriate that, since federal and state governments will reap considerable benefit from the efficient practice of medicine, they help fund efforts to achieve that goal.

## GOAL 3—FOR THE SYSTEM: IMPROVE COST, QUALITY, AND LIFE EXPECTANCY

Cost and quality must be considered together. We do not want to reduce cost and have quality suffer. We should strive to reduce costs while *improving* quality. How does that happen? We've already stated that we waste a third of our health-care dollars, about $1 trillion per year.[26] With passage of the ACA, states are saddled with the added yearly cost associated with expand-ing Medicaid, estimated to be $135 billion.[27] If we could save just 15 percent of the waste—$150 billion—we could cover the ACA with no increase in taxes.

We must work to further address chronic disease, reduce hospital read-missions and unnecessary admissions, and cut down on unnecessary visits to the emergency department. These reforms, while improving patient out-comes, could reduce the cost of care by an additional 10 percent.[28]

US life expectancy is forty-third in the world.[29] There is no reason—other than an unwillingness to take on hard work—that we should not be in the top ten.

## CHAPTER SUMMARY

- Most Americans can agree on goals for our health-care system.
- *Goal 1—For the people: Coverage for all with accessible, affordable, adequate health care*

- Coverage is very different from access and means that a person has insurance—either public or private.
- A person has access in health care if that person can see the right medical practitioner at the right time and in the right place. The "right place" can be e-mail or video and is *not* the emergency department for colds and sore throats. But access remains a challenge in many rural *and* urban settings. Note that *coverage*, frequently confused with access, means that the person has health insurance. Remember it this way: perfect coverage with no access occurs in West Texas, where patients have a Medicare card and no doctor to see them; perfect access with no coverage occurs in every emergency room, where patients can be seen and receive care but have no insurance to help pay for it.
- Most people consider 2–5 percent of income to be affordable for their out-of-pocket health-insurance costs. We're nowhere near that level of affordability.
- We face an ongoing discussion about what constitutes "adequate" health care. Regardless, US health care can't mean whatever care anyone wants, because it would be too pricey.

- *Goal 2—For practitioners: Pay based on quality, and eliminate hassles*

  - The most sensible way to deliver value-based care is to pay physicians a salary. Care should be hassle-free, including a well-functioning EHR system. Physicians now spend only 55 percent of their time in direct care of patients.

- *Goal 3—For the system: Improve cost, quality, and life expectancy*

  - We do not want to reduce cost at the expense of quality. As costs come down, insurance becomes more affordable. Our most pointed attack should be on chronic disease. Reducing readmissions, unnecessary admissions, and emergency-department visits could improve the health of those with chronic disease and reduce the total cost of care by 10 percent.
  - The US life expectancy is forty-third in the world. There is no reason—other than hard work—that we should not be in the top ten.

## Chapter Twenty

# Myth: There Is No Health-Care System That Will Work for the United States

Given the deep, philosophical divisions in our political system in the United States—not to mention the long, entrenched political clout of the health-care sector—it may seem that our health-care system is so flawed that it will be impossible to fix it. Should we give up? Not a chance.

## A REMINDER OF HOW WE GOT HERE

We believe there's a clear road map that can point us toward a future fix. But first, let's review the history. Modern health care in the United States had a major change in the late 1940s when health insurance was provided as a benefit by employers. Then, in the mid-1960s, amid a great deal of "social conscience," we added government programs for those who needed help: The Medicare program covered those over sixty-five who were retired or retiring. The Medicaid system was set up to help those who did not work— children, pregnant women, the disabled, and those covered by Medicare who could not pay even the relatively small Medicare coinsurance. Eventually, as an outgrowth of other long-term care, Medicaid began to cover low-income nursing-home patients.[1] All of this made sense until the cost of health care increased and health insurance became impossible for businesses to cover. This was, and remains today, the case for many small businesses. Medicaid was not designed to cover people between ages nineteen and sixty-four, because the thinking was that these people could work, and their health insurance would be provided through the employer. But that didn't happen.

And now we are faced with a large number of uninsured, most of whom work but are employed by businesses that don't help cover health insurance.

This hodgepodge of health-care programs can hardly be considered a "system"—certainly nothing that works together, anyway. Why, for example, is Medicare a federal program while Medicaid is a program shared between the federal and state governments? We see at least two reasons: First, each state has its own way of dealing with assistance programs. Some are generous, and some are less generous, depending on each state's revenue and spending priorities. Some of these policies result from attitudes of general dislike of government, particularly the federal government. This dislike seems to go hand in hand with less aid to those with low incomes. It would be unlikely that those "less generous" states would be in favor of a more generous program that took all control away from the states, handing it over to the federal government.

The second reason is a practical one: states must balance their budgets; the federal government does not have this restriction. Therefore, any major increase in spending, and health care for all, will require plenty of increased spending and must be led by the federal government.

Niccolò Machiavelli said, "There is nothing more difficult to plan, more doubtful of success, nor more dangerous to manage than a new system. For the initiator has the enmity of all who would profit by the preservation of the old institution and merely lukewarm defenders in those who gain by the new ones."[2] And this is likely why major change in our health-care system has been resisted: there will be big winners and big losers. Nobody wants to lose, so few at the top are overly eager to change.

And so we are left with a health-care *nonsystem* that doesn't work at all. The parts of our nonsystem were created long ago, under conditions that no longer apply today. So what can we propose instead?

## AN EVENTUAL SOLUTION FOR THE UNITED STATES: MEDICARE FOR ALL OR A SINGLE SAFETY NET?

### Medicare for All

It's worthwhile taking the time to discuss possible long-term solutions to our health-care system. But we must recognize that no solution can be created and implemented immediately; change will be incremental—as discussed in chapter 18. Many in the United States are throwing around the phrase *Medi-*

*care for all.* What do they mean by it? Well, Medicare for all would mean different things to different people, and so it's not always clear which model people are talking about. Some models would consist of Medicare coverage while prohibiting the addition of private insurance[3]—similar to the Canadian model. Other models would allow private insurance[4]—like the UK model, the single safety net. The reality is that in the United States we value capitalism and competition. And our politicians pay attention to the powerful insurance lobby. The idea of rendering the entire private health-insurance industry illegal is likely a nonstarter if we're looking for workable change. In a country where you can pay extra to get more legroom on a flight, where you can pay a premium to drive in a faster freeway lane, and where you can even pay a fee to skip the lines at Disney World, it's hard to imagine that we'd ever agree that people shouldn't be allowed to pay extra for extras in health care.

## The Single Safety Net

The eventual solution, in our view, is a *single safety net* of health care, where government-funded health care is available to all. In our proposed system, private insurance isn't banned, and those who want to purchase additional coverage are free to purchase it. Employers can continue to offer private insurance for their employees, but it would be in addition to a baseline of coverage that everyone would already have. And there would be no tax breaks for employers, the way there are today.

There's precedent for this, of course: the public-school system is a single safety net of education. After all, all children in the United States have the right to a free, government-provided education. But if parents have the desire—and resources—they can enroll their child in private school. We envision a similar system for health care: those who do not have insurance would have basic coverage from the single safety net.

The health-care single-safety-net model is in operation in nearly every country in the world. We'd like to take credit for offering a unique, novel concept, but we can't. But does it really matter to us that every other country has this kind of system? Not really. The United States shouldn't adopt this solution *because* it's used around the world, but its widespread use suggests that something's working and that it's something worth considering.

So let's consider it.

The United Kingdom has a health-care single safety net supplemented with the availability of private insurance. Virtually all UK residents use the

National Health Service (NHS) to meet their basic health-care needs. The government funds the NHS just as the US government funds current Medicare. But about 10 percent of the UK population uses private health insurance that they add to their basic coverage provided by the NHS. Why do they do this? Through private insurance, they may be able to get appointments more quickly or easily, and they may have a wider variety of drugs covered by their plan.[5]

The United Kingdom does not have a single-payer system. The term *single-payer* is thrown around in the health-care debate, often as a shorthand for *universal health care* or *publicly funded health care*. But here's an important distinction: in *single-payer* health care only one entity, the government, pays for health care. This would mean that in a single-payer system, private health insurance doesn't exist. Canada is the only major country using a true single-payer health-care system. While Canadians can and do use private insurance to pay for some things—like dental work, optometry, and some prescription medication not covered by the basic government plan—for all intents and purposes, Canadians receive all of their health care from a solely government-funded system, without the help of private insurance.

Creating a single safety net offers choice: Those who want to pay out of pocket, or via private insurance, for a costly treatment that may not be effective in most patients would be free to do so. Far be it from anyone to stop them. The difference is that taxpayers wouldn't have to cover the more expensive choice.

The challenge, of course, is how to make any true system work. Let's start with current Medicare, which is really popular among the patients it covers.[6] It pays for all services pretty much without restriction. Any future true health system, no matter what it is called, will not be able to cover all services. Policy makers would have to make difficult, thoughtful decisions about how to direct resources toward treatments that are most likely to be effective—and likely deny spending on more questionable types of care. Some may call this rationing; others may call it rational. Such decisions would be informed by cost-effectiveness analysis or, more simply, working to pay for limited resources. So far in the United States we haven't much acted like we realize we *do* have limited resources—but the fact is, *we have limited resources*. There are other priorities that must be funded besides health care. And in the single safety net, tests and treatments that are proven to provide bang for their buck would be funded rather than those that are long shots or wasteful. As part of this process, it would be crucial that we obtain citizen input to help ensure the decisions are as fair and representative as possible. But rationing will be a major sticking point and may stand in the way of serious change. Furthermore, Medicare today barely pays providers sufficiently. Physician and hospital payment will be another major sticking point in negotiations as we work to modify health care and actually have a system.

Of course, one massive question is how to pay for it. Given the variation in proposals and the likelihood that none of them will not be enacted tomorrow, it is not worthwhile to dwell on actual numbers. The interested reader can investigate current calculations.[7] One thing is for sure: we will have to decrease the cost of health care, and even so, it will require more money. Covering millions more people is more expensive than leaving them uninsured and more likely to die.

As we think about it, there just is no other workable long-term fix other than what we've proposed. We've intentionally called this a *single safety net* rather than a *single-payer* system, which has been labeled "socialized medicine." We don't call public school *socialized education*; yet, as a country, we think it's a good idea that all students, regardless of their resources, can enroll. And this health-care program would substantively be no different. We have seen earlier in the book that noninterference—"just letting the market work"—isn't going to get us where we need to go; although even if the status quo is maintained, at the very least efforts to better inform consumers must be made. But in the end, if we want better health care, we need a true system. One way to get that system is to allow state experimentation to find a model, prove it's workable, and scale it nationally.

## HOW DO WE GET FROM HERE TO THERE? GIVE THE STATES A CHANCE

The federal government could promote state health reform. The state programs would be models for eventual national adoption. In this case, perhaps states could develop various approaches to a single safety net—or test different ideas altogether. State health-care reform is both an end and a means: As states begin to improve coverage and reform the health-care systems within their borders, the numbers of uninsured will be reduced—an important improvement in and of itself. However, and equally important, state experiments will help determine which programs work and which don't, making the odds for success much improved. State initiatives in all areas of policy have traditionally provided impetus for innovation.[8]

In its fullest sense, during this "laboratory phase," the United States could end up with fifty different state plans for managing health care, which is not likely to be desirable. More likely, though, a few states will demonstrate successes that will then inform the development of a federal program—and that will likely be replicated by other states. We've seen this happen before: health reforms in Massachusetts in the mid-2000s provided the outline for the Affordable Care Act, which became national law just a few years later. Clearly if states are to be models for the whole country, any eventual unifying federal program would need to provide pathways to move from state approaches to a national one.

In 2007, senators Jeff Bingaman (Democrat, representing New Mexico) and George Voinovich (Republican, representing Ohio) introduced the Health Partnership Act, and a similar bill won bipartisan support in the House.[9] The HPA, as it is known, authorized grants to individual states and groups of states with the idea of spurring health-policy innovation. Each applicant's program would need to increase health-care coverage, improve health-care quality and efficiency, and use information technology to improve health-care infrastructure. A bipartisan commission would create yearly targets for coverage, quality, cost, and information technology and decide which states to fund. At the end of the that period, that commission would report to Congress whether states were meeting the grant-mandated goals and would recommend future action Congress should take concerning broader reforms.

But the bills never became law. They were moving through both the Senate and the House when then-presidential candidate John Edwards proposed his own plan for national health-care reform, quickly followed by fellow Democratic candidates Hillary Clinton and Barack Obama. Fast forward to the present, and we may well have come full circle. Attempts at overall federal reform have failed, and we could again look to the states.

Of course, states couldn't address these issues in a vacuum, given the federal intersection with health policy through ERISA, Medicare, and Medicaid, among other issues. Nevertheless, promoting state-based reform has the potential to inform national discussions when and if the political will for reform emerges.

## OKAY, BUT WHEN?

But when can we expect real health-care reform to occur? We think it likely that the economic will to reform the system will arise only when the price of health care is so intolerable for individuals, employers, and the nation that action becomes a necessity. As we learned from the American Health Care Act in 2017, it is possible for a political movement to begin with the president and capture the support of a large number of legislators. It is either economic or political conditions (or both) that will sufficiently incentivize the change of our troubled health care nonsystem. Hopefully next time the stars align for a change it will mean affordable, accessible, efficient, and effective medical care—and health care—for all Americans.

## CHAPTER SUMMARY

- One thing's for sure: We don't really have a health care "system" now. Rather, it's many systems cobbled together, over many years, without real planning.
- What's the eventual solution? No plan would be implementable tomorrow; even so, it's worth considering answers as we move into the future.
- *Medicare for all* has referred to a number of different health-care models. Some proposals ban private insurance, while others accept it. Banning private insurance is likely be a nonstarter in the United States, because some will want to add to the basic coverage they would receive.
- A better idea is a *single safety net* where basic government-funded health care is available to all and those who want to purchase additional coverage are also free to do so. There's precedent for this in the United States in the public-school system—a program nobody's denigrating as "socialized education." A way to get there is to allow states to experiment with their own health-care overhauls to identify and prove a workable concept that can be applied nationally.
- The single safety net is akin to the United Kingdom's health-care system, where 10 percent of the population supplements their basic care using private insurance. Essentially all countries other than the United States have a version of this, the only outlier being Canada, where a truly single-payer system provides government-funded health care, with private insurance only covering what the basic plan does not.

- Major change will likely not occur in our health-care system until the price of health care is so intolerable for individuals, employers, and the nation that action *must* occur. Additionally, this type of change won't be possible without a president who is committed to changing the health of our nation and without a majority of legislators who agree. Whether the impetus is economic or political, Americans will have to come together to act if we want to reform our troubled health-care *nonsystem*.

# Final Words

We hope that after reading this book the current problems facing the US health-care system and the possible ways to deal with them will be more understandable. Surely the "myths" by now are busted. In so doing, we need to get past the negative mindset in which we believe that nothing will work, that health care is irrevocably broken, but instead proceed toward positive solutions. The important decisions will ultimately be left to the people, and not just through their elected officials but also through direct participation in discussions about what is best for the nation. We can do this together.

> Your assumptions are your windows on the world. Scrub them off every once in a while, or the light won't come in.
>
> —Attributed to Isaac Asimov

> For me, it is far better to grasp the Universe as it really is than to persist in delusion, however satisfying and reassuring.
>
> —Carl Sagan[1]

> Any fool can know. The point is to understand.
>
> —Attributed to Albert Einstein

> Everyone is entitled to his own opinion but not to his own facts.
>
> —Attributed to Daniel Patrick Moynihan

# Notes

## PREFACE

1. "Poll: Health Care Remains Top Priority for Americans," News, Harvard School of Public Health (website), 2017, https://www.hsph.harvard.edu/news/hsph-in-the-news/poll-health-care-priority-for-americans/.

2. Katherine Wilson, "National Health Spending Passes $10,000 per Person, and We Should Be Concerned," *California Health Care Foundation Blog*, June 11, 2018, https://www.chcf.org/blog/national-health-spending-passes-10000-and-we-should-be-concerned/.

3. "The World Factbook," CIA.gov, accessed March 22, 2019, https://www.cia.gov/library/publications/the-world-factbook/rankorder/2102rank.html.

4. Joshua Cohen, "Troublesome News: Numbers of Uninsured on the Rise," *Forbes*, July 6, 2018, https://www.forbes.com/sites/joshuacohen/2018/07/06/troublesome-news-numbers-of-uninsured-on-the-rise/#534f7864309f.

5. Arthur Garson and Carolyn L. Engelhard, *Health Care Half-Truths: Too Many Myths, Not Enough Reality* (Lanham, MD: Rowman & Littlefield, 2007).

## 1. MYTH: US HEALTH CARE IS THE BEST IN THE WORLD

1. J. Michael McGinnis, Pamela Williams-Russo, and James R. Knickman, "The Case for More Active Policy Attention to Health Promotion," *Health Affairs* 21, no. 2 (2002): 78–93, https://www.healthaffairs.org/doi/pdf/10.1377/hlthaff.21.2.78.

2. John J. Goldman, "Men's Death Rate Higher in Harlem than Bangladesh," *LA Times*, January 18, 1990, http://articles.latimes.com/1990-01-18/news/mn-336_1_death-rate.

3. "Social Determinants of Health: Key Concepts," World Health Organization (website), https://www.who.int/social_determinants/thecommission/finalreport/key_concepts/en/, accessed October 19, 2018.

4. Lindsey Cook, "Why Black Americans Die Younger," US News and World Report, January 5, 2015, https://www.usnews.com/news/blogs/data-mine/2015/01/05/black-americans-have-fewer-years-to-live-heres-why.

5. Steven Reinberg, "Life Expectancy Tied to Education," *Washington Post*, March 11, 2008, http://www.washingtonpost.com/wp-dyn/content/article/2008/03/11/AR2008031100925 .html.

6. Alice Park, "Nearly Half of US Deaths Can Be Prevented with Lifestyle Changes," *Time*, May 1, 2014, http://time.com/84514/nearly-half-of-us-deaths-can-be-prevented-with-lifestyle-changes/.

7. Ashish P. Thakrar, Alexandra D. Forrest, Mitchell G. Maltenfort, and Christopher B. Forrest, "Child Mortality in the US And 19 OECD Comparator Nations: A 50-Year Time-Trend Analysis," *Health Affairs* 37, no.1 (2018): 140–49, doi:10.1377/hlthaff.2017.0767.

8. Kate Devlin, "AAAS: Living Near Trees 'Makes People Live Longer and Feel Happi-er,'" *The Telegraph*, February 13, 2009, https://www.telegraph.co.uk/news/earth/earthnews/ 4612176/AAAS-Living-near-trees-makes-people-live-longer-and-feel-happier.html.

9. Andrew W. Wilper, Steffie Woolhandler, Karen E. Lasser, Danny McCormick, David H. Bor, and David U. Himmelstein, "Health Insurance and Mortality in US Adults," *American Journal of Public Health* 99, no. 12 (2009): 2289–95, doi:10.2105/AJPH.2008.157685.

10. Nicholette Zeliadt, "Live Long and Proper: Genetic Factors Associated with Increased Longevity Identified," *Scientific American*, July 1, 2010, https://www.scientificamerican.com/ article/genetic-factors-associated-with-increased-longevity-identified/.

11. "Ten Great Public Health Achievements—United States, 1900–1999," *Morbidity and Mortality Weekly Report*, April 2, 1999, https://www.cdc.gov/mmwr/preview/mmwrhtml/ 00056796.htm.

12. Suzanne Lacasse and Farrokh Nadim, "Learning to Live with Geohazards: From Re-search to Practice," in *Geotechnical Special Publication*, ed. American Society of Civil Engi-neers (Reston, VA: American Society of Civil Engineers, 2011), 64–116, doi:10.1061/ 41183(418)4, originally presented at the Georisk 2011 conference, June 2011, Atlanta, Geor-gia.

13. The 2017 data is pulled from "The World Factbook," Central Intelligence Agency (web-site), https://www.cia.gov/library/publications/the-world-factbook/rankorder/2091rank.html, accessed March 23, 2018.

14. Rafael Lozano, Mohsen Naghavi, Kyle Foreman, Stephen Lim, Kenji Shibuya, Victor Aboyans, Jerry Abraham, Timothy Adair, Rakesh Aggarwal, and Stephanie Y. Ahn, "Global and Regional Mortality from 235 Causes of Death for 20 Age Groups in 1990 and 2010: A Systematic Analysis for the Global Burden of Disease Study 2010," *The Lancet* 380, no. 9859 (2012): 2095–2128, doi:10.1016/S0140-6736(12)61728-0.

15. Brieanna Davis, "Teenage Pregnancy: The United States Has the Highest Rate of by . . ." presentation published online at Prezi, updated January 26, 2016, https://prezi.com/ 95qchcyfgoyp/teenage-pregnancy-the-united-states-has-the-highest-rate-of/.

16. Catherine L. Kothari, Rajib Paul, Ben Dormitorio, Fernando Ospina, Arthur James, Deb Lenz, Kathleen Baker, Amy Curtis, and James Wiley, "The Interplay of Race, Socioeconomic Status and Neighborhood Residence upon Birth Outcomes in a High Black Infant Mortality Community," *SSM—Population Health* 2 (2016): 859–67, retrieved from https://www.ncbi. nlm.nih.gov/pmc/articles/PMC5757914/, doi:10.1016/j.ssmph.2016.09.011.

17. Alice Chen, Emily Oster, and Heidi Williams, "Why Is Infant Mortality Higher in the United States than in Europe?" *American Economic Journal: Economic Policy* 8, no. 2 (2016): 89–124, retrieved from https://www.ncbi.nlm.nih.gov/pmc/articles/PMC4856058/, doi:10.1257 /pol.20140224.

18. Catherine L. Kothari, Rajib Paul, Ben Dormitorio, Fernando Ospina, Arthur James, Deb Lenz, Kathleen Baker, Amy Curtis, and James Wiley, "The Interplay of Race, Socioeconomic Status and Neighborhood Residence upon Birth Outcomes in a High Black Infant Mortality Community," *SSM—Population Health* 2 (2016): 859–67, retrieved from https://www.ncbi.nlm.nih.gov/pmc/articles/PMC5757914/, doi:10.1016/j.ssmph.2016.09.011.

19. Institute of Medicine, "The Effectiveness of Prenatal Care," in *Preventing Low Birthrate* (Washington, DC: National Academies Press, 1985), ch. 6, retrieved from https://www.ncbi.nlm.nih.gov/books/NBK214461/.

20. Alice Chen, Emily Oster, and Heidi Williams, "Why Is Infant Mortality Higher in the United States than in Europe?" *American Economic Journal: Economic Policy* 8, no. 2 (2016): 89–124, available online at https://www.ncbi.nlm.nih.gov/pmc/articles/PMC4856058/, doi:10.1257/pol.20140224.

21. "New Study: U.S. Performs Worst on Potentially Preventable Death Rates Compared to France, Germany, and the U.K.; U.S. Also Improving at Slowest Pace," Commonwealth Fund (website), August 29, 2012, http://www.commonwealthfund.org/~/media/files/news/news-releases/2012/aug/nolte-release-final-82712.pdf.

22. GBD 2015 Healthcare Access and Quality Collaborators, "Healthcare Access and Quality Index Based on Mortality from Causes Amenable to Personal Health Care in 195 Countries and Territories, 1990–2015: A Novel Analysis from the Global Burden of Disease Study 2015," *The Lancet* 390, no. 10091 (2017): 231–66, https://www.thelancet.com/journals/lancet/article/PIIS0140-6736(17)30818-8/fulltext, doi:10.1016/S0140-6736(17)30818-8.

23. "New Study: U.S. Performs Worst on Potentially Preventable Death Rates Compared to France, Germany, and the U.K.; U.S. Also Improving at Slowest Pace," Commonwealth Fund (website), August 29, 2012, http://www.commonwealthfund.org/~/media/files/news/news-releases/2012/aug/nolte-release-final-82712.pdf.

24. The Institute for Health Metrics and Evaluation, "America's Ranking on Amenable Mortality Is an Embarrassment," Physicians for a National Health Program (website), May 18, 2017, http://pnhp.org/blog/2017/05/19/americas-ranking-on-amenable-mortality-is-an-embarrassment/.

# 2. MYTH: IN MANY WAYS, US HEALTH CARE IS CHEAPER THAN OTHER COUNTRIES'

1. Gerard F. Anderson, Uwe E. Reinhardt, Peter S. Hussey, and Varduhi Petrosyan, "It's The Prices, Stupid: Why the United States Is So Different from Other Countries," *Health Affairs* 22, no. 3 (2003): 89–105, https://www.healthaffairs.org/doi/pdf/10.1377/hlthaff.22.3.89.

2. Rabah Kamal and Cynthia Cox, "How Do Healthcare Prices and Use in the U.S. Compare to Other Countries?" Peterson-Kaiser Health System Tracker, May 8, 2018, https://www.healthsystemtracker.org/chart-collection/how-do-healthcare-prices-and-use-in-the-u-s-compare-to-other-countries/#item-the-average-price-of-an-mri-in-the-u-s-is-significantly-higher-than-in-comparable-countries_2018.

3. Jacob Funk Kirkegaard, "The True Levels of Government and Social Expenditures in Advanced Economies," Peterson Institute for International Economics (website), March 2015, https://piie.com/publications/pb/pb15-4.pdf.

4. Ibid.

5. "NHE-Fact-Sheet," Centers for Medicare and Medicaid Services (website), last modified February 20, 2019, https://www.cms.gov/research-statistics-data-and-systems/statistics-trends-and-reports/nationalhealthexpenddata/nhe-fact-sheet.html.

6. "National Health Expenditures 2017 Highlights," Centers for Medicare and Medicaid Services (website), https://www.cms.gov/research-statistics-data-and-systems/statistics-trends-and-reports/nationalhealthexpenddata/downloads/highlights.pdf, accessed February 11, 2018.

7. "How Does Health Spending in the U.S. Compare to Other Countries?" Henry J. Kaiser Family Foundation (website), https://www.kff.org/slideshow/health-spending-in-the-u-s-as-compared-to-other-countries-slideshow/, accessed October 10, 2018.

8. Bradley Sawyer and Cynthia Cox, "How Does Health Spending in the U.S. Compare to Other Countries?" Peterson-Kaiser Health System Tracker, December 7, 2018, https://www.healthsystemtracker.org/chart-collection/health-spending-u-s-compare-countries/#item-relative-size-wealth-u-s-spends-disproportionate-amount-health.

9. Susan Brink, "What Country Spends the Most (And Least) on Health Care per Person?" NPR, April 20, 2017, https://www.npr.org/sections/goatsandsoda/2017/04/20/524774195/what-country-spends-the-most-and-least-on-health-care-per-person.

10. Stuart Silverstein, "This Is Why Your Drug Prescriptions Cost So Damn Much," *Mother Jones*, October 21, 2016, https://www.motherjones.com/politics/2016/10/drug-industry-pharmaceutical-lobbyists-medicare-part-d-prices/.

11. Visit the National Institute for Health and Care Excellence online at https://www.nice.org.uk/.

12. Jacqueline R. Fox, "Medicare Should, but Cannot, Consider Cost: Legal Impediments to a Sound Policy," *Buffalo Law Review* 53, no. 2 (2005): 577–633, retrieved from https://scholarcommons.sc.edu/cgi/viewcontent.cgi?article=2098&context=law_facpub.

13. David U. Himmelstein, Miraya Jun, Reinhard Busse, Karine Chevreul, Alexander Geissler, Patrick Jeurissen, Sarah Thomson, Marie-Amelie Vinet, and Steffie Woolhandler, "A Comparison of Hospital Administrative Costs in Eight Nations: US Costs Exceed All Others by Far," *Health Affairs* 33, no. 9 (2014): 1586–94, https://www.healthaffairs.org/doi/full/10.1377/hlthaff.2013.1327, doi:10.1377/hlthaff.2013.1327.

14. Gerard F. Anderson, Uwe E. Reinhardt, Peter S. Hussey, and Varduhi Petrosyan, "It's The Prices, Stupid: Why the United States Is So Different from Other Countries," *Health Affairs* 22, no. 3 (2003): 89–105, https://www.healthaffairs.org/doi/pdf/10.1377/hlthaff.22.3.89.

15. Organisation for Economic Co-operation and Development, "Number of Practicing Physicians per 1,000 Population, 2014," International Health Care System Profiles (website), Commonwealth Fund, 2016, https://international.commonwealthfund.org/stats/number_practicing_physicians/; Organisation for Economic Co-operation and Development, "Total Curative (Acute) Care Beds, per 1,000 Population, 2014," International Health Care System Profiles (website), Commonwealth Fund, 2016, https://international.commonwealthfund.org/stats/acute_care_hospital_beds/.

16. Donald M. Berwick and Andrew D. Hackbarth, "Eliminating Waste in US Health Care," *Journal of the American Medical Association* 307, no. 14 (2012): 1513–16, doi:10.1001/jama.2012.362.

17. Jacob Funk Kirkegaard, "The True Levels of Government and Social Expenditures in Advanced Economies," Peterson Institute for International Economics (website), March 2015, https://piie.com/publications/pb/pb15-4.pdf.

18. Elizabeth H. Bradley, Benjamin R. Elkins, Jeph Herrin, and Brian Elbel, "Health and Social Services Expenditures: Associations with Health Outcomes," *BMJ Quality & Safety* 20, no. 10 (2011): 826–31, doi:10.1136/bmjqs.2010.048363.

# 3. MYTH: THE UNITED STATES WASTES ONE IN EVERY TEN MEDICAL-CARE DOLLARS

1. Steve Sternberg and Geoff Dougherty, "Are Doctors Exposing Heart Patients to Unnecessary Cardiac Procedures?" US News and World Report, February 11, 2015, https://www.usnews.com/news/articles/2015/02/11/are-doctors-exposing-heart-patients-to-unnecessary-cardiac-procedures.

2. Donald M. Berwick and Andrew D. Hackbarth, "Eliminating Waste in US Health Care," *Journal of the American Medical Association* 307, no. 14 (2012): 1513–16, doi:10.1001/jama.2012.362.

3. Ryan Whitacker, "How Much Universal Healthcare Would Cost in the US," Decision-Data.org, November 11, 2015, https://decisiondata.org/news/how-much-single-payer-uhc-would-cost-usa/.

4. Eva-Julia Weyler and Afschin Gandjour, "Empirical Validation of Patient versus Population Preferences in Calculating QALYs," *Health Services Research* 46, no. 5 (2011): 1562–74, doi:10.1111/j.1475-6773.2011.01268.x.

5. David U. Himmelstein, Miraya Jun, Reinhard Busse, Karine Chevreul, Alexander Geissler, Patrick Jeurissen, Sarah Thomson, Marie-Amelie Vinet, and Steffie Woolhandler, "A Comparison of Hospital Administrative Costs in Eight Nations: US Costs Exceed All Others by Far," *Health Affairs* 33, no. 9 (2014): 1586–94, https://www.heailthaffairs.org/doi/full/10.1377/hlthaff.2013.1327, doi:10.1377/hlthaff.2013.1327.

6. Manuela Tobias, "Comparing Administrative Costs for Private Insurance and Medicare," PolitiFact (website), September 20, 2017, http://www.politifact.com/truth-o-meter/statements/2017/sep/20/bernie-s/comparing-administrative-costs-private-insurance-a/.

7. Donald M. Berwick and Andrew D. Hackbarth, "Eliminating Waste in US Health Care," *Journal of the American Medical Association* 307, no. 14 (2012): 1513–16, doi:10.1001/jama.2012.362.

8. Scott E. Hadland, Maxwell S. Krieger, and Brandon David Lewis Marshall, "Industry Payments to Physicians for Opioid Products, 2013–2015," *American Journal of Public Health* 107, no. 9 (2017): 1493–95, doi:10.2105/AJPH.2017.303982.

9. Alix Spiegel, "How the Modern Patient Drives Up Health Costs," NPR, October 12, 2009, https://www.npr.org/templates/story/story.php?storyId=113664923.

10. Eve A. Kerr, Jeffrey T. Kullgren, and Sameer D. Saini, "Choosing Wisely: How to Fulfill the Promise in the Next 5 Years," *Health Affairs* 36, no. 11 (2017): 2012–18, doi:10.1377/hlthaff.2017.0953.

11. Scott E. Hadland, Maxwell S. Krieger, and Brandon David Lewis Marshall, "Industry Payments to Physicians for Opioid Products, 2013–2015," *American Journal of Public Health* 107, no. 9 (2017): 1493–95, doi:10.2105/AJPH.2017.303982.

12. Quoted by melly in "Assessing 'Waste' in Medical Care," *American Medical Care* (blog), September 2010, http://americanmedicalcare.blogspot.com/2010/09/assessing-waste-in-medical-care.html.

13. Quoted by Michael D. Miller in "More on Evidence Based Medicine," *Dr. Miller's Health Policy and Communications Blog*, March 6, 2008, http://www.healthpolcom.com/blog/2008/03/06/more-on-evidence-based-medicine/.

14. "Medicare Program: Additional Actions Needed to Improve Eligibility Verification of Providers and Suppliers," US Government Accountability Office (website), June 25, 2015, GAO-15-448, https://www.gao.gov/products/GAO-15-448.

15. William J. Rudman, John S. Eberhardt, William Pierce, and Susan Hart-Hester, "Healthcare Fraud and Abuse," *Perspectives in Health Information Management* 16, no. 6 (2009): 1g, retrieved from https://www.ncbi.nlm.nih.gov/pmc/articles/PMC2804462/.

16. Michael D. Miller, "More on Evidence Based Medicine," *Dr. Miller's Health Policy and Communications Blog*, March 6, 2008, http://www.healthpolcom.com/blog/2008/03/06/more-on-evidence-based-medicine/.

17. Ibid.

18. "Medicare Program: Additional Actions Needed to Improve Eligibility Verification of Providers and Suppliers," US Government Accountability Office (website), June 25, 2015, GAO-15-448, https://www.gao.gov/products/GAO-15-448.

19. Michael D. Miller, "More on Evidence Based Medicine," *Dr. Miller's Health Policy and Communications Blog*, March 6, 2008, http://www.healthpolcom.com/blog/2008/03/06/more-on-evidence-based-medicine/.

20. Gerard F. Anderson, Uwe E. Reinhardt, Peter S. Hussey, and Varduhi Petrosyan, "It's The Prices, Stupid: Why the United States Is So Different from Other Countries," *Health Affairs* 22, no. 3 (2003): 89–105, https://www.healthaffairs.org/doi/pdf/10.1377/hlthaff.22.3.89.

21. Anna Medaris Miller, "5 Common Preventable Medical Errors," US News and World Report, March 30, 2015, https://health.usnews.com/health-news/patient-advice/slideshows/5-common-preventable-medical-errors.

22. Colleen K. McIlvennan, Zubin J. Eapen, and Larry A. Allen, "Hospital Readmissions Reduction Program," *Circulation* 131, no. 20 (2015): 1796–1803, retrieved from https://www.ncbi.nlm.nih.gov/pmc/articles/PMC4439931/, doi:10.1161/CIRCULATIONAHA.114.010270.

23. Craig Thomas, "A Structured Home Visit Program by Non-licensed Healthcare Personnel Can Make a Difference in the Management and Readmission of Heart Failure Patients," *Journal of Hospital Administration* 3, no. 3 (2014): 1–6, http://www.sciedu.ca/journal/index.php/jha/article/view/3473/2256, doi:10.5430/jha.v3n3p1.

24. S. Craig Thomas, Robert A. Greevy, and Arthur Garson, "Effect of Grand-Aides Nurse Extenders on Readmissions and Emergency Department Visits in Medicare Patients with Heart Failure," *American Journal of Cardiology* 121, no. 11 (2018): 1336–42, https://www.ajconline.org/article/S0002-9149(18)30248-0/pdf, doi:10.1016/J.AMJCARD.2018.02.012.

25. Rachael B. Zuckerman, Steven H. Sheingold, E. John Orav, Joel Ruhter, and Arnold M. Epstein, "Readmissions, Observation, and the Hospital Readmissions Reduction Program," *New England Journal of Medicine* 374, no. 16 (2016): 1543–51, https://www.nejm.org/doi/10.1056/NEJMsa1513024, doi:10.1056/NEJMsa1513024.

26. Cristina Boccuti, "Aiming for Fewer Hospital U-turns: The Medicare Hospital Readmission Reduction Program," Henry J. Kaiser Family Foundation (website), March 10, 2017, https://www.kff.org/medicare/issue-brief/aiming-for-fewer-hospital-u-turns-the-medicare-hospital-readmission-reduction-program/.

## 4. MYTH: MOST MEDICAL-CARE DOLLARS ARE SPENT IN THE LAST SIX MONTHS OF LIFE

1. Juliette Cubanski, Tricia Neuman, Shannon Griffin, and Anthony Damico, "Medicare Spending at the End of Life: A Snapshot of Beneficiaries Who Died in 2014 and the Cost of

Their Care; Findings," Henry J. Kaiser Family Foundation (website), July 14, 2016, https://www.kff.org/report-section/medicare-spending-at-the-end-of-life-findings/.

2. Ibid.

3. Eric B. French, Jeremy McCauley, Maria Aragon, Pieter Bakx, Martin Chalkley, Stacey H. Chen, Bent J. Christensen, et al., "End-of-Life Medical Spending in Last Twelve Months of Life Is Lower than Previously Reported," *Health Affairs* 36, no. 7 (2017): 1211–17, https://www.healthaffairs.org/doi/full/10.1377/hlthaff.2017.0174, doi:10.1377/hlthaff.2017.0174.

4. Ibid.

5. Liz Hamel, Bryan Wu, and Mollyann Brodie, "Views and Experiences with End-of-Life Medical Care in the U.S.," report, Henry J. Kaiser Family Foundation, April 2017, http://files.kff.org/attachment/Report-Views-and-Experiences-with-End-of-Life-Medical-Care-in-the-US.

6. Angie Drobnic Holan, "PolitiFact's Lie of the Year: 'Death Panels,'" PolitiFact, December 18, 2009, https://www.politifact.com/truth-o-meter/article/2009/dec/18/politifact-lie-year-death-panels/.

7. PRNewswire-USNewswire, "Nearly Two-Thirds of Americans Don't Have Living Wills—Do You?" American College of Emergency Physicians (website), March 21, 2016, http://newsroom.acep.org/2016-03-21-Nearly-Two-Thirds-of-Americans-Dont-Have-Living-Wills-Do-You.

8. Alan R. Weil and Rachel Dolan, eds., "Improving Care at the End of Life: A Report of the Aspen Institute Health Strategy Group," foreword by Kathleen Sebelius and Tommy G. Thompson, Aspen Institute Health Strategy Group, 2016, https://assets.aspeninstitute.org/content/uploads/2017/02/AHSG-Report-Improving-Care-at-the-End-of-Life.pdf.

9. Ibid.

10. Ibid.

11. Martha Hostetter and Sarah Klein, "Improving Care at the End of Life," Commonwealth Fund (website), June–July 2012, http://www.commonwealthfund.org/publications/newsletters/quality-matters/2012/june-july/in-focus.

12. DailyCaring editorial team, "Make Sure End-of-Life Wishes Are Honored with a POLST," DailyCaring, http://dailycaring.com/polst-why-your-older-adult-may-need-one/, accessed March 29, 2018.

13. S. Craig Thomas, Robert A. Greevy Jr., and Arthur Garson Jr., "Effect of Grand-Aides Nurse Extenders on Readmissions and Emergency Department Visits in Medicare Patients with Heart Failure," *American Journal of Cardiology* 121, no. 11 (2018): 1336–42, https://www.ajconline.org/article/S0002-9149(18)30248-0/fulltext, doi:10.1016/j.amjcard.2018.02.012.

14. Scott A. Murray, Marilyn Kendall, Kirsty Boyd, and Aziz Sheikh, "Illness Trajectories and Palliative Care," *BMJ* 330, no. 7498 (2005): 1007–11, retrieved from https://www.ncbi.nlm.nih.gov/pmc/articles/PMC557152/, doi:10.1136/bmj.330.7498.1007.

15. "What Is Palliative Care?" Medical Encyclopedia, MedlinePlus, last updated January 28, 2019, https://medlineplus.gov/ency/patientinstructions/000536.htm.

16. Caroline Stephens, Elizabeth Halifax, Nhat Bui, Sei J. Lee, Charlene Harrington, Janet Shim, and Christine Ritchie, "Provider Perspectives on the Influence of Family on Nursing Home Resident Transfers to the Emergency Department: Crises at the End of Life," *Current Gerontology and Geriatrics Research* (2015):893062, doi:10.1155/2015/893062.

17. Robert Kreisman, "$28.5 Million Jury Verdict for Nursing Home's Failure to Timely Transfer Resident to Hospital," *Chicago Nursing Home Lawyers Blog*, January 25, 2018, https://www.robertkreisman.com/nursing-home-lawyer/2018/01/25/28-5-million-jury-verdict-nursing-homes-failure-timely-transfer-resident-hospital/.

18. Liz Hamel, Bryan Wu, and Mollyann Brodie, "Views and Experiences with End-of-Life Medical Care in the U.S.," report, Henry J. Kaiser Family Foundation, April 2017, http://files. kff.org/attachment/Report-Views-and-Experiences-with-End-of-Life-Medical-Care-in-the-US.

19. Jaya K. Rao, Lynda A. Anderson, Feng-Chang Lin, and Jeffrey P. Laux, "Completion of Advance Directives among U.S. Consumers," *American Journal of Preventative Medicine* 46, no. 1 (2014): 65–70, https://www.ajpmonline.org/article/S0749-3797(13)00521-7/fulltext, doi: 10.1016/j.amepre.2013.09.008.

20. Alexis Dallara, Alan Carver, and Eli Diamond, "Aggressive Medical Care and the End of Life (EOL) in Glioblastoma (GBM): The 5-Year Memorial Sloan-Kettering Cancer Center (MSKCC) Experience (P7.273)," *American Academy of Neurology* 82 (2014): P7.273, http://n. neurology.org/content/82/10_Supplement/P7.273.

21. Pippa Hawley, "Barriers to Access to Palliative Care," *Palliative Care* 10 (2017): 1178224216688887, retrieved from https://www.ncbi.nlm.nih.gov/pmc/articles/PMC5398324/, doi:10.1177/1178224216688887.

22. Ibid.

23. Penelope Wang, "Cutting the High Cost of End-of-Life Care," *Money*, December 12, 2012, http://time.com/money/2793643/cutting-the-high-cost-of-end-of-life-care/.

24. The Medicare Payment Advisory Commission, "Chapter 12: Hospice Services," in *Report to the Congress: Medicare Payment Policy*, March 15, 2017, 315–42, http://www.medpac. gov/docs/default-source/reports/mar17_medpac_ch12.pdf.

25. Ryan Holeywell, "Experts Urge Expanded Use of Advance Directives for End-of-Life Care," TMC News, April 23, 2018, http://www.tmc.edu/news/2018/04/end-of-life-care-advance-directives/.

# 5. MYTH: THE UNITED STATES CONSISTENTLY PROVIDES HIGH-QUALITY MEDICAL CARE

1. Institute of Medicine, *Crossing the Quality Chasm: A New Health System for the 21st Century* (Washington, DC: National Academies Press, 2001), doi:10.17226/10027.

2. Bridget A. Stewart, Susan Fernandes, Elizabeth Rodriguez-Huertas, and Michael Landzberg, "A Preliminary Look at Duplicate Testing Associated with Lack of Electronic Health Record Interoperability for Transferred Patients," *Journal of the American Medical Informatics Association* 17, no. 3 (2010): 341–44, https://www.ncbi.nlm.nih.gov/pmc/articles/PMC 2995707/, doi:10.1136/jamia.2009.001750.

3. Sabrina Tavernise, "Black Americans See Gains in Life Expectancy," *New York Times*, May 9, 2015, https://www.nytimes.com/2016/05/09/health/blacks-see-gains-in-life-expectancy .html.

4. Frances P. Boscoe, Kevin A. Henry, Recinda L. Sherman, and Christopher J. Johnson, "The Relationship between Cancer Incidence, Stage, and Poverty in the United States Recommended Citation," *Epidemiology and Biostatistics Faculty Scholarship* (2015), https:// scholarsarchive.library.albany.edu/cgi/viewcontent.cgi?article=1002&context=epi_fac_ scholar.

5. Gopal K. Singh and Mohammad Siahpush, "Widening Rural-Urban Disparities in All-Cause Mortality and Mortality from Major Causes of Death in the USA, 1969–2009," *Journal of Urban Health* 91, no. 2 (2014): 272–92, retrieved from https://www.ncbi.nlm.nih.gov/pmc/ articles/PMC3978153/, doi:10.1007/s11524-013-9847-2.

6. John J. Goldman, "Men's Death Rate Higher in Harlem than Bangladesh," *LA Times*, January 18, 1990, http://articles.latimes.com/1990-01-18/news/mn-336_1_death-rate.

7. Michelle M. Mello, Amitahb Chandra, Atul A. Gawande, and David M. Studdert, "National Costs of the Medical Liability System," *Health Affairs* 29, no. 9 (2010): 1569–77, retrieved from https://www.ncbi.nlm.nih.gov/pmc/articles/PMC3048809/, doi:10.1377/hlth aff.2009.0807.

8. Niki Carver and John E. Hipskind, "Medical Error," *StatPearls*, last updated October 27, 2018, retrieved from https://www.ncbi.nlm.nih.gov/books/NBK430763/.

9. Cara Livernois, "Only 18 Percent of Clinical Recommendations Are Evidence-Based," *AI in Healthcare*, June 22, 2017, https://www.clinical-innovation.com/topics/analytics-quality/only-18-clinical-recommendations-are-evidence-based.

10. Debra S. Echt, Philip R. Liebson, L. Brent Mitchell, Robert W. Peters, Dulce Obias-Manno, Allan H. Barker, Daniel Arensberg, et al., "Mortality and Morbidity in Patients Receiving Encainide, Flecainide, or Placebo: The Cardiac Arrhythmia Suppression Trial," *New England Journal of Medicine* 324, no. 12 (1991): 781–88, https://www.nejm.org/doi/10.1056/NEJM199103213241201, doi:10.1056/NEJM199103213241201.

11. "So, No Rescue Breaths with CPR, Right?" EMS Safety Services (website), February 15, 2016, http://www.emssafetyservices.com/2016/02/15/so-no-rescue-breaths-with-cpr-right/.

12. Vinay Prasad, Andrae Vandross, Caitlin Toomey, Michael Cheung, Jason Rho, Steven Quinn, Satish Jacob Chacko, et al., "A Decade of Reversal: An Analysis of 146 Contradicted Medical Practices," *Mayo Clinic Proceedings* 88, no. 8 (2013): 790–98, https://www.mayoclinicproceedings.org/article/S0025-6196(13)00405-9/fulltext, doi:10.1016/j.mayocp.20 13.05.012.

13. Ibid.

14. The Action to Control Cardiovascular Risk in Diabetes Study Group, "Effects of Intensive Glucose Lowering in Type 2 Diabetes," *New England Journal of Medicine* 358, no. 24 (2008): 2545–59, https://www.nejm.org/doi/10.1056/NEJMoa0802743, doi:10.1056/NEJMoa 0802743.

15. Henry Bodkin, "Patients Treated by Older Doctors More Likely to Die, New Research Indicates," *Telegraph*, May 16, 2017, https://www.telegraph.co.uk/news/2017/05/16/patients-treated-older-doctors-likely-die-new-research-indicates/; Yusuke Tsugawa, Joseph P. Newhouse, Alan M. Zaslavsky, Daniel M. Blumenthal, and Anupam B. Jena, "Physician Age and Outcomes in Elderly Patients in Hospital in the US: Observational Study," *BMJ* 357 (2017): j1797, https://www.bmj.com/content/357/bmj.j1797, doi:10.1136/BMJ.J1797; Lucy Pasha-Robinson, "Older Doctors Linked to Higher Death Rates among Patients, Study Finds," *The Independent*, May 16, 2017, https://www.independent.co.uk/news/health/older-doctors-linked-higher-death-rates-patients-bmj-study-a7739576.html.

16. Steve Sternberg and Geoff Dougherty, "Are Doctors Exposing Heart Patients to Unnecessary Cardiac Procedures?" US News and World Report, February 11, 2015, https://www.usnews.com/news/articles/2015/02/11/are-doctors-exposing-heart-patients-to-unnecessary-cardiac-procedures.

17. Alberto J. Montero, "Guidelines Are Essential to Improving Clinical Outcomes in Breast Cancer Patients," *Breast Cancer Research and Treatment* 153, no. 1 (2015): 1–2, retrieved from https://link.springer.com/article/10.1007/s10549-015-3526-9, doi:10.1007/s10549-015-3526-9.

18. Paul G. Shekelle, "Clinical Practice Guidelines: What's Next?" *Journal of the American Medical Association* 320, no. 8 (2018): 757, doi:10.1001/jama.2018.9660.

19. Ana-Catarina Pinho-Gomes, Luis Azevedo, Jung-Min Ahn, Seung-Jung Park, Taye H. Hamza, Michael E. Farkouh, Patrick W. Serruys, et al., "Compliance with Guideline-Directed

Medical Therapy in Contemporary Coronary Revascularization Trials," *Journal of the American College of Cardiology* 71, no. 6 (2018): 591–602, http://www.onlinejacc.org/content/71/6/591, doi:10.1016/J.JACC.2017.11.068.

20. "2016 National Healthcare Quality and Disparities Report," Agency for Healthcare Research and Quality, June 2017, available from https://www.ahrq.gov/research/findings/nhqrdr/nhqdr16/index.html.

21. Mitchell H. Katz, Deborah Grady, and Rita F. Redberg, "Undertreatment Improves, but Overtreatment Does Not," *JAMA Internal Medicine* 173, no. 2 (2013): 93, doi:10.1001/jamainternmed.2013.2361.

22. "2016 National Healthcare Quality and Disparities Report," Agency for Healthcare Research and Quality, June 2017, available from https://www.ahrq.gov/research/findings/nhqrdr/nhqdr16/index.html.

23. Christopher Stomberg, Margaret Albaugh, Saul Shiffman, and Neeraj Sood, "A Cost-Effectiveness Analysis of Over-the-Counter Statins," *American Journal of Managed Care* 22, no. 5 (2016): e294–303, http://www.ncbi.nlm.nih.gov/pubmed/27266585.

24. Gary Claxton, Larry Levitt, Matthew Rae, and Bradley Sawyer, "Increases in Cost-Sharing Payments Continue to Outpace Wage Growth," Peterson-Kaiser Health System Tracker, June 15, 2018, https://www.healthsystemtracker.org/brief/increases-in-cost-sharing-payments-have-far-outpaced-wage-growth/.

# 6. MYTH: CONSUMERS MAKE THE BEST DECISIONS ABOUT THEIR MEDICAL CARE

1. Arthur "Tim" Garson Jr., "One of Many Problems with Short-Term Insurance Plans: Consumers Can't Understand Them," *STAT*, March 6, 2018, https://www.statnews.com/2018/03/06/short-term-health-insurance-consumers/.

2. Lynn D. Silver, Shu Wen Ng, Suzanne Ryan-Ibarra, Lindsey Smith Taillie, Marta Induni, Donna R. Miles, Jennifer M. Poti, and Barry M. Popkin, "Changes in Prices, Sales, Consumer Spending, and Beverage Consumption One Year after a Tax on Sugar-Sweetened Beverages in Berkeley, California, US: A Before-and-After Study," *PLOS Medicine* 14, no. 4 (2017): e1002283, https://journals.plos.org/plosmedicine/article?id=10.1371/journal.pmed.1002283, doi:10.1371/journal.pmed.1002283.

3. Arthur "Tim" Garson, Stephen H. Linder, and Ryan Holeywell, "The Nation's Pulse: The Texas Medical Center's Customer & Physician Survey," slides of survey findings, Texas Medical Center, 2017, https://www.tmc.edu/health-policy/wp-content/uploads/sites/5/2017/09/2017NationsPulsePresentation.pdf.

4. Jonah Comstock, "Prediction: 24 Million Will Use Diabetes Apps by 2018," *MobiHealthNews*, March 24, 2014, https://www.mobihealthnews.com/31313/prediction-24-million-will-use-diabetes-apps-by-2018.

5. Bianca DiJulio, Jamie Firth, and Mollyann Brodie, "Kaiser Health Tracking Poll: August 2015," Henry J. Kaiser Family Foundation (website), August 20, 2015, https://www.kff.org/health-costs/poll-finding/kaiser-health-tracking-poll-august-2015/.

6. E. Goldstein and J. Fyock, "Reporting of CAHPS Quality Information to Medicare Beneficiaries," *Health Services Research* 36, no. 3 (2001): 477–88, available for download from https://www.ncbi.nlm.nih.gov/pmc/articles/PMC1089238/.

7. Ibid.

8. "Safe Surgery Checklist Use," *Medicare.gov*, accessed March 22, 2019, https://www. medicare.gov/hospitalcompare/hospital-safe-surgery-checklist.html; find the Automatic Readability Checker we used for our analysis at http://www.readabilityformulas.com/free-readability-formula-tests.php.

9. Rajender Agarwal, Olena Mazurenko, and Nir Menachemi, "High-Deductible Health Plans Reduce Health Care Cost and Utilization, Including Use of Needed Preventive Services," *Health Affairs* 36, no. 10 (2017): 1762–68, doi:10.1377/hlthaff.2017.0610.

10. Kaitlyn Houseman, "10 Most Popular Physician Rating and Review Sites," *GroupOne Revenue Cycle Blog*, June 1, 2017, http://www.grouponehealthsource.com/blog/10-most-popular-physician-rating-and-review-sites.

11. Visit Healthgrades online at https://www.healthgrades.com/.

12. From a search performed for "Houston, TX" and "TMH Physician Associates PLLC" at Medicaid.gov's website, Physician Compare, https://www.medicare.gov/physiciancompare/ #profile&loc=HOUSTON, TX&lat=29.7601927&lng=-95.3693896&flow=default&paging= 1&keyword=TMH Physician Associates PLLC&dist=15&pid=4486711744&loctype=c, accessed October 27, 2018.

13. Anna Almendrala, "Many Doctors Who Face Malpractice Suits Are Serial Offenders," *HuffPost Life*, January 29, 2016, https://www.huffpost.com/entry/doctors-malpractice-research_n_56a94bece4b05e4e37033d00.

14. Review the New York State Department of Health's Cardiac Surgery and PCI (Angioplasty) Reports and Forms online at https://www.health.ny.gov/health_care/consumer_ information/cardiac_surgery/.

15. For US News and World Report's Best Hospitals by Regional Ranking, visit https:// health.usnews.com/best-hospitals/area.

16. Karen Pollitz, Jennifer Tolbert, and Rosa Ma, "Survey of Health Insurance Marketplace Assister Programs," Executive Summary, Henry J. Kaiser Family Foundation (website), July 15, 2014, https://www.kff.org/health-reform/report/survey-of-health-insurance-marketplace-assister-programs/.

# 7. MYTH: PREVENTIVE CARE SAVES MONEY

1. Louis Jacobson, "Barack Obama Says Preventive Care 'Saves Money,'" PolitiFact, February 10, 2012, https://www.politifact.com/truth-o-meter/statements/2012/feb/10/barack-obama/barack-obama-says-preventive-care-saves-money/.

2. Louise B. Russell, "Preventing Chronic Disease: An Important Investment, but Don't Count on Cost Savings," *Health Affairs* 28, no. 1 (2009): 42–45, https://www.healthaffairs.org/ doi/full/10.1377/hlthaff.28.1.42, doi:10.1377/hlthaff.28.1.42.

3. Arthur Garson Jr., "Prevention Is Good Medicine but It's Not a Fiscal Panacea," op-ed, *USA Today*, February 13, 2008.

4. Joshua T. Cohen, Peter J. Neumann, and Milton C. Weinstein, "Does Preventive Care Save Money? Health Economics and the Presidential Candidates," *New England Journal of Medicine* 358, no. 7 (2008): 661–63, http://www.nejm.org/doi/pdf/10.1056/NEJMp0708558.

5. Quoted in "Willard Gaylin: Ethics, Biology, and Economics," *Moyers*, September 20, 1988, https://billmoyers.com/content/willard-gaylin/.

6. Al Lewis and Vik Khanna, "Corporate Wellness Programs Lose Money," *Harvard Business Review*, October 15, 2015, https://hbr.org/2015/10/corporate-wellness-programs-lose-money.

7. Natasha Singer, "Health Plan Penalty Ends at Penn State," *New York Times*, September 19, 2013, https://www.nytimes.com/2013/09/19/business/after-uproar-penn-state-suspends-penalty-fee-in-wellness-plan.html.

8. Tom Emerick and Al Lewis, "The Danger of Wellness Programs: Don't Become the Next Penn State," *Harvard Business Review*, August 20, 2013, https://hbr.org/2013/08/attention-human-resources-exec.

9. Ibid.

10. Jon K. Maner, Andrea Dittmann, Andrea L. Meltzer, and James K. McNulty, "Implications of Life-History Strategies for Obesity," *Proceedings of the National Academy of Sciences of the United States of America* 114, no. 32 (2017): 8517–22, https://www.pnas.org/content/114/32/8517, doi:10.1073/pnas.1620482114.

11. Paul K. Whelton, Jiang He, Lawrence J. Appel, Jeffrey A. Cutler, Stephen Havas, Theodore A. Kotchen, Edward J. Roccella, et al., "Primary Prevention of Hypertension: Clinical and Public Health Advisory from the National High Blood Pressure Education Program," *Journal of the American Medical Association* 288, no. 15 (2002): 1882, https://jamanetwork.com/journals/jama/article-abstract/195419, doi:10.1001/jama.288.15.1882.

12. Stephen E. Fienberg and David C. Hoaglin, eds., *Selected Papers of Frederick Mosteller* (New York: Springer New York, 2006).

13. Paul K. Whelton, Jiang He, Lawrence J. Appel, Jeffrey A. Cutler, Stephen Havas, Theodore A. Kotchen, Edward J. Roccella, et al., "Primary Prevention of Hypertension: Clinical and Public Health Advisory from the National High Blood Pressure Education Program," *Journal of the American Medical Association* 288, no. 15 (2002): 1882, https://jamanetwork.com/journals/jama/article-abstract/195419, doi:10.1001/jama.288.15.1882.

14. Micah Berman, Rob Crane, Eric Seiber, and Mehmet Munur, "Estimating the Cost of a Smoking Employee," *Tobacco Control* 23, no. 5 (2014): 428–33, doi:10.1136/tobaccocontrol-2012-050888.

15. Ibid.

16. Kathleen Michon, "Tobacco Litigation: History and Recent Developments," Nolo (website), https://www.nolo.com/legal-encyclopedia/tobacco-litigation-history-and-development-32202.html, accessed October 28, 2018.

17. "Master Settlement Agreement," Public Health Law Center (website), http://publichealthlawcenter.org/topics/tobacco-control/tobacco-control-litigation/master-settlement-agreement, accessed October 28, 2018.

18. James R. Baumgardner, Linda T. Bilheimer, Mark B. Booth, William J. Carrington, Noelia J. Duchovny, and Ellen C. Werble, "Cigarette Taxes and the Federal Budget: Report from the CBO," *New England Journal of Medicine* 367, no. 22 (2012): 2068–70, https://www.nejm.org/doi/full/10.1056/NEJMp1210319, doi:10.1056/NEJMp1210319.

19. Mike Patton, "U.S. Health Care Costs Rise Faster than Inflation," *Forbes*, June 29, 2015, https://www.forbes.com/sites/mikepatton/2015/06/29/u-s-health-care-costs-rise-faster-than-inflation/#33996b8e6fa1.

20. Brian D. Giacomino, Peter Cram, Mary Vaughan-Sarrazin, Yunshu Zhou, and Saket Girotra, "Association of Hospital Prices for Coronary Artery Bypass Grafting with Hospital Quality and Reimbursement," *American Journal of Cardiology* 117, no. 7 (2016): 1101–6, https://www.ajconline.org/article/S0002-9149(16)30013-3/fulltext, doi:10.1016/j.amjcard.2016.01.004.

21. Elise Cruz, "Crutchfield Employee Wellness Program Now Includes Local Produce," *Charlottesville Tomorrow*, July 5, 2015, https://www.cvilletomorrow.org/articles/crutchfield-csa.

# 8. MYTH: THE UNITED STATES WILL NOT RATION MEDICAL CARE

1. Ryan Holeywell, "How High Will Drug Prices Climb?" TMC News, March 9, 2018, http://www.tmc.edu/news/2018/03/how-high-will-drug-prices-climb/.

2. Marah Noel Short, Thomas A. Aloia, and Vivian Ho, "The Influence of Complications on the Costs of Complex Cancer Surgery," *Cancer* 120, no. 7 (2014): 1035–41, doi:10.1002/cncr.28527.

3. Ryan Holeywell, "How High Will Drug Prices Climb?" TMC News, March 9, 2018, http://www.tmc.edu/news/2018/03/how-high-will-drug-prices-climb/.

4. Arthur Garson Jr. and Carolyn L. Engelhard, "You Can't Have It All," *Governing*, July 14, 2009, http://www.governing.com/topics/health-human-services/You-Cant-Have-It.html.

5. Christopher R. Blagg, "The Early History of Dialysis for Chronic Renal Failure in the United States: A View from Seattle," *American Journal Kidney Diseases* 49, no. 3 (2007): 482–96, https://www.ajkd.org/article/S0272-6386(07)00116-3/fulltext, doi:10.1053/j.ajkd .2007.01.017.

6. Jonathan Oberlander, Theodore Marmor, and Lawrence Jacobs, "Rationing Medical Care: Rhetoric and Reality in the Oregon Health Plan," *Canadian Medical Association Journal* 164, no. 11 (2001): 1583–87, http://www.cmaj.ca/content/164/11/1583.long.

7. Bob DiPrete and Darren D. Coffman, "A Brief History of Health Services Prioritization in Oregon," Oregon Health Association (website), March 2007, available at https://www.acupunctureresearch.org/assets/docs/C2017/PrioritizationHistory_Coffman.pdf.

8. Jonathan Oberlander, Theodore Marmor, and Lawrence Jacobs, "Rationing Medical Care: Rhetoric and Reality in the Oregon Health Plan," *Canadian Medical Association Journal* 164, no. 11 (2001): 1583–87, http://www.cmaj.ca/content/164/11/1583.long.

9. Gary L. Albrecht, "Rationing Health Care to Disabled People," *Sociology of Health and Illness* 23, no. 5 (2001): 654–77, retrieved from https://onlinelibrary.wiley.com/doi/pdf/10.1111/1467-9566.00270, doi:10.1111/1467-9566.00270.

10. Jonathan Oberlander, Theodore Marmor, and Lawrence Jacobs, "Rationing Medical Care: Rhetoric and Reality in the Oregon Health Plan," *Canadian Medical Association Journal* 164, no. 11 (2001): 1583–87, http://www.cmaj.ca/content/164/11/1583.long.

11. Eric Fruits, "The Oregon Health Plan: A 'Bold Experiment' that Failed," *SSRN Electronic Journal*, September 21, 2010, available for download at https://papers.ssrn.com/sol3/papers.cfm?abstract_id=1680047.

12. Karen Donelan, Catherine M. DesRoches, Robert S. Dittus, and Peter Buerhaus, "Perspectives of Physicians and Nurse Practitioners on Primary Care Practice," *New England Journal of Medicine* 368, no. 20 (2013): 1898–1906, https://www.nejm.org/doi/10.1056/NEJMsa1212938, doi:10.1056/NEJMsa1212938.

13. Anne Dunkelberg, "Child Friendly? How Texas' Policy Choices Affect Whether Children Get Enrolled and Stay Enrolled in Medicaid and CHIP," Center for Public Policy Priorities, revised 2008, http://library.cppp.org/files/3/CHILD FRIENDLY 0208forweb.pdf.

14. The Kaiser Commission on Medicaid and the Uninsured, "Barriers to Medicaid Enrollment for Low-Income Seniors: Focus Group Findings," Henry J. Kaiser Family Foundation (website), January 2002, http://files.kff.org/attachment/Barriers-to-Medicaid-Enrollment-for-Seniors-Findings-from-10-Focus-Groups-with-Low-Income-Seniors-Report.

15. Jonathan Oberlander, Theodore Marmor, and Lawrence Jacobs, "Rationing Medical Care: Rhetoric and Reality in the Oregon Health Plan," *Canadian Medical Association Journal* 164, no. 11 (2001): 1583–87, http://www.cmaj.ca/content/164/11/1583.long.

16. "High Deductible Health Plan (HDHP)," Glossary, HealthCare.gov, https://www.healthcare.gov/glossary/high-deductible-health-plan/, accessed October 6, 2018.

17. "Who We Are," National Institute for Health and Care Excellence (website), https://www.nice.org.uk/about/who-we-are, accessed February 16, 2018.

18. "NICE Technology Appraisal Guidance," National Institute for Health and Care Excellence (website), https://www.nice.org.uk/About/What-we-do/Our-Programmes/NICE-guidance/NICE-technology-appraisal-guidance, accessed October 9, 2018.

19. Ibid.

20. Peter Singer, "Why We Must Ration Health Care," *New York Times*, July 15, 2009, https://www.nytimes.com/2009/07/19/magazine/19healthcare-t.html.

21. Paul R. Womble, James E. Montie, Zaojun Ye, Susan M. Linsell, Brian R. Lane, and David C. Miller, "Contemporary Use of Initial Active Surveillance among Men in Michigan with Low-Risk Prostate Cancer," *European Urology* 67, no. 1 (2015): 44–50, doi:10.1016/j.eururo.2014.08.024.

22. Anne Underwood and Sarah Arnquist, "Healthcare Abroad: France," *Prescriptions* (blog), *New York Times*, September 11, 2009, https://prescriptions.blogs.nytimes.com/2009/09/11/health-care-abroad-france/.

23. Ashish Jha, "The People's Hospital: Cost, Transparency, and Hospital Care in the Middle of China," *An Ounce of Evidence: Health Policy* (blog), January 10, 2014, https://blogs.sph.harvard.edu/ashish-jha/2014/01/10/the-peoples-hospital-cost-transparency-and-hospital-care-in-the-middle-of-china/.

24. John M. Eisenberg, "Clinical Economics: A Guide to the Economic Analysis of Clinical Practices," *Journal of the American Medical Association* 262, no. 20 (1989): 2879, doi:10.1001/jama.1989.03430200123038.

25. Govind Persad, Alan Wertheimer, and Ezekiel J. Emanuel, "Principles for Allocation of Scarce Medical Interventions," *The Lancet* 373, no. 9661 (2009): 423–31, doi:10.1016/S0140-6736(09)60137-9.

26. Ibid.

27. Dave Anderson, "Sports of the Times; 'I'll Try to Make Up for Stuff,'" *New York Times*, July 12, 1995, https://www.nytimes.com/1995/07/12/sports/sports-of-the-times-i-ll-try-to-make-up-for-stuff.html.

28. Govind Persad, Alan Wertheimer, and Ezekiel J. Emanuel, "Principles for Allocation of Scarce Medical Interventions," *The Lancet* 373, no. 9661 (2009): 423–31, doi:10.1016/S0140-6736(09)60137-9.

29. Arthur Garson Jr. and Carolyn L. Engelhard, "You Can't Have It All," *Governing*, July 14, 2009, http://www.governing.com/topics/health-human-services/You-Cant-Have-It.html.

## 9. MYTH: THE UNITED STATES FACES
## A DANGEROUS SHORTAGE OF DOCTORS

1. "Recent Studies and Reports on Physician Shortages in the US," Association of American Medical Colleges, October 2012, https://www.aamc.org/download/100598/data/.

2. IHS Markit, "The Complexities of Physician Supply and Demand: Projections from 2015 to 2030; Final Report," Association of American Medical Colleges, February 28, 2017, https://aamc-black.global.ssl.fastly.net/production/media/filer_public/a5/c3/a5c3d565-14ec-48fb-974b-99fafaeecb00/aamc_projections_update_2017.pdf.

3. Arthur Garson, "New Systems of Care Can Leverage the Health Care Workforce: How Many Doctors Do We Really Need?" *Academic Medicine* 88, no. 12 (2013): 1817–21, doi:10.1097/ACM.0000000000000006.

4. Organisation for Economic Co-operation and Development, *The Looming Crisis in the Health Workforce: How Can OECD Countries Respond?* (Paris: OECD Publishing, 2008), http://www.oecd.org/els/health-systems/41509236.pdf.

5. Merritt Hawkins team, "2017 Survey of Physician Appointment Wait Times," Merritt Hawkins (website), September 22, 2017, https://www.merritthawkins.com/news-and-insights/thought-leadership/survey/survey-of-physician-appointment-wait-times/.

6. Ibid.

7. "US Medical School Enrollment Up 25% since 2002," news release, Association of American Medical Colleges (website), May 25, 2017, https://news.aamc.org/press-releases/article/enrollment-05252017/.

8. "Section and Table Listing," in "Survey of Resident/Fellow Stipends and Benefits Report, 2016–2017," Association of American Medical Colleges, November 2016, 1–3, https://www.aamc.org/download/471828/data/2016stipendsurveyreportfinal.pdf.

9. Ramin LaLezari, "Why Does Medicare Pay Resident Salaries?" *KevinMD*, November 16, 2014, https://www.kevinmd.com/blog/2014/11/medicare-pay-resident-salaries.html.

10. "Table 1. Resident/Fellow Current Year Actual Stipends Nationwide, Dollar Change and Percent Change from 2014–2015, Academic Year 2016–2017," in "Survey of Resident/Fellow Stipends and Benefits Report, 2016–2017," Association of American Medical Colleges, November 2016, 7, https://www.aamc.org/download/471828/data/2016stipendsurveyreportfinal.pdf.

11. "New Grad RN Salaries," Salaries, Glassdoor (website), updated February 27, 2019, https://www.glassdoor.com/Salaries/new-grad-rn-salary-SRCH_KO0,11.htm.

12. Amy Orciari Herman, "Female, but Not Male, Physicians Work Fewer Hours When They Have Children," *New England Journal of Medicine Journal Watch*, August 22, 2017, https://www.jwatch.org/fw113237/2017/08/22/female-not-male-physicians-work-fewer-hours-when-they, doi:10.1056/NEJM-JW.FW113237.

13. Daniël van Hassel, Lud van der Velden, Dinny de Bakker, and Ronald Batenburg, "Age-Related Differences in Working Hours among Male and Female GPs: An SMS-Based Time Use Study," *Human Resources for Health* 15, no. 1 (2017): 84, https://www.ncbi.nlm.nih.gov/pmc/articles/PMC5735885/, doi:10.1186/s12960-017-0258-4.

14. IHS Markit, "The Complexities of Physician Supply and Demand: Projections from 2015 to 2030; Final Report," Association of American Medical Colleges, February 28, 2017, https://aamc-black.global.ssl.fastly.net/production/media/filer_public/a5/c3/a5c3d565-14ec-48fb-974b-99fafaeecb00/aamc_projections_update_2017.pdf.

15. National Center for Health Workforce Analysis, "National and Regional Projections of Supply and Demand for Primary Care Practitioners: 2013–2025," Health Resources and Services Administration, November 2016, https://bhw.hrsa.gov/sites/default/files/bhw/health-workforce-analysis/research/projections/primary-care-national-projections2013-2025.pdf.

16. Melanie Swan, Sacha Ferguson, Alice Chang, Elaine Larson, and Arlene Smaldone, "Quality of Primary Care by Advanced Practice Nurses: A Systematic Review," *International Journal for Quality in Health Care* 27, no. 5 (2015): 396–404, https://academic.oup.com/intqhc/article/27/5/396/2357352, doi:10.1093/intqhc/mzv054.

17. "Where Can Nurse Practitioners Work without Physician Supervision?" *Nursing Blog*, Simmons University, October 25, 2016, https://onlinenursing.simmons.edu/nursing-blog/nurse-practitioners-scope-of-practice-map/.

18. Robert Hoyt, "The Future of EHRs—Trends Driving EHR Adoption," Practice Fusion (website), https://www.practicefusion.com/health-informatics-practical-guide-page-8/, accessed February 16, 2018.

19. Mark Mather, "Fact Sheet: Aging in the United States," Population Reference Bureau (website), January 13, 2016, http://www.prb.org/Publications/Media-Guides/2016/aging-united states-fact-sheet.aspx.

20. "When I'm 64: How Boomers Will Change Health Care," American Hospital Association (website), May 2007, https://www.aha.org/system/files/content/00-10/070508-boomer report.pdf.

21. IHS Markit, "The Complexities of Physician Supply and Demand: Projections from 2015 to 2030; Final Report," Association of American Medical Colleges, February 28, 2017, https://aamc-black.global.ssl.fastly.net/production/media/filer_public/a5/c3/a5c3d565-14ec-48fb-974b-99fafaeecb00/aamc_projections_update_2017.pdf.

22. T. Gosden, Frode Forland, Ivar Sonobo Kristiansen, Matt Sutton, Brenda Leese, Antonio Giuffrida, M. Sergison, and L. Pedersen, "Capitation, Salary, Fee-for-Service and Mixed Systems of Payment: Effects on the Behaviour of Primary Care Physicians," *Cochrane Database of Systematic Review* 3, no. 3 (2000), CD002215, doi:10.1002/14651858.CD002215.

23. Ateev Mehrotra and Allan Prochazka, "Improving Value in Health Care: Against the Annual Physical," *New England Journal of Medicine* 373, no. 16 (2015): 1485–87, doi:10.1056/NEJMp1507485; Robert Hoyt, "The Future of EHRs—Trends Driving EHR Adoption," Practice Fusion (website), https://www.practicefusion.com/health-informatics-practical-guide-page-8/, accessed February 16, 2018.

24. Arthur Garson, "Perspective: Leveraging the Health Care Workforce; What Do We Need and What Educational System Will Get Us There?" *Academic Medicine* 86, no. 11 (2011): 1448–53, doi:10.1097/ACM.0b013e318230588b.

25. Anna Leach, "Task Shifting Explained: A Viable Solution to Health Worker Shortage?" Global Development Professionals Network, *The Guardian*, May 12, 2014, https://www.theguardian.com/global-development-professionals-network/2014/may/12/task-shifting-health-development-shortage.

26. Doug Olson, "Primary Care Doctors May No Longer Be Needed," *KevinMD*, December 24, 2012, https://www.kevinmd.com/blog/2012/12/primary-care-doctors-longer-needed.html.

27. Catherine DesRoches, Peter Buerhaus, Robert Dittus, and Karen Donelan, "Primary Care Workforce Shortages and Career Recommendations from Practicing Clinicians," *Academic Medicine* 90, no. 5 (2015): 671–77, doi:10.1097/ACM.0000000000000591.

28. Mahesh Goenka, Rakesh Kochhar, D. N. Reddy, and Prateek Sharma, "Endoscopy Training: Indian Perspective," *Journal of Digestive Endoscopy* 5, no. 4 (2014): 135, retrieved from https://www.researchgate.net/publication/273181150_Endoscopy_training_Indian_per spective, doi:10.4103/0976-5042.150658; Srinivas Marmamula, Rohit C. Khanna, Konegari

Shekhar, and Gullapalli N. Rao, "Outcomes of Cataract Surgery in Urban and Rural Population in the South Indian State of Andhra Pradesh: Rapid Assessment of Visual Impairment (RAVI) Project," ed. Islam FMA, *PLoS One* 11, no. 12 (2016): e0167708, https://journals.plos.org/plosone/article?id=10.1371/journal.pone.0167708, doi:10.1371/journal.pone.0167708.

29. Arthur Garson, Donna M. Green, Lia Rodriguez, Richard Beech, and Christopher Nye, "A New Corps of Trained Grand-Aides Has the Potential to Extend Reach of Primary Care Workforce and Save Money," *Health Affairs* 31, no. 5 (2012): 1016–21, https://www.healthaffairs.org/doi/full/10.1377/hlthaff.2011.0859, doi:10.1377/hlthaff.2011.0859.

30. S. Craig Thomas, Robert A. Greevy, and Arthur Garson Jr., "Effect of Grand-Aides Nurse Extenders on Readmissions and Emergency Department Visits in Medicare Patients with Heart Failure," *American Journal of Cardiology* 121, no. 11 (2018): 1336–42, https://www.ajconline.org/article/S0002-9149(18)30248-0/pdf, doi:10.1016/j.amjcard.2018.02.012; Arthur Garson, "Grand-Aides and Health Policy: Reducing Readmissions Cost-Effectively," *Health Affairs Blog*, October 29, 2014, https://www.healthaffairs.org/do/10.1377/hblog20141029.041916/full/.

31. J. Michael Mcginnis, Pamela Williams-Russo, and James R. Knickman, "The Case for More Active Policy Attention to Health Promotion," *Health Affairs* 21, no. 2 (2002): 78–93, https://www.healthaffairs.org/doi/pdf/10.1377/hlthaff.21.2.78.

32. Amelia Goodfellow, Jusus G. Ulloa, Patrick T. Dowling, Efrain Talamantes, Somil Chheda, and Gerardo Moreno, "Predictors of Primary Care Physician Practice Location in Underserved Urban or Rural Areas in the United States: A Systematic Literature Review," *Academic Medicine* 91, no. 9 (2016): 1313–21, doi:10.1097/ACM.0000000000001203; Dawn Goodlove, "Greener Pastures: Needing Rural Doctors, Iowa Grows Its Own (And Pays for the Training)," *Medicine Iowa* (Summer 2016), https://medcom.uiowa.edu/medicine/greener-pastures/. For information on repayment of loans to pay for medical care, visit the Health Resources and Services Administration at https://nhsc.hrsa.gov/loanrepayment/.

33. Anne Cantrell, "MSU Study Finds Nurse Practitioners More Likely than Medical Doctors to Work in Rural Areas," Montana State University (website), January 14, 2016, http://www.montana.edu/news/15928/msu-study-finds-nurse-practitioners-more-likely-than-medical-doctors-to-work-in-rural-areas.

34. Sarah Collins, "Primary Care Shortages: Strengthening This Sector Is Urgently Needed, Now and in Preparation for Healthcare Reform," *American Health and Drug Benefits* 5, no. 1 (2012): 40–47, https://www.ncbi.nlm.nih.gov/pmc/articles/PMC4046463/.

# 10. MYTH: THE CURRENT MALPRACTICE SYSTEM PROTECTS PATIENTS

1. David Goguen, "Medical Negligence," AllLaw.com, http://www.alllaw.com/articles/nolo/medical-malpractice/negligence.html, accessed October 8, 2018.

2. Byren Warnken, "77% of Medical Malpractice Jury Trials Result in Defense Verdicts," Injury Lawyer Database Maryland (website), September 8, 2013, https://www.injurylawyerdatabase.com/blog/2013/09/77-of-medical-malpractice-jury-trials-result-in-defense-verdicts/.

3. To find these statistics on medical malpractice damages and more, see David Goguen, "State-by-State Medical Malpractice Damages Caps," Nolo (website), https://www.nolo.com/legal-encyclopedia/state-state-medical-malpractice-damages-caps.html, accessed February 14, 2018.

4. Dennis Thompson, "Fewer Medical Malpractice Lawsuits Succeed, but Payouts Are Up," CBS News, March 28, 2017, https://www.cbsnews.com/news/medical-malpractice-lawsuits-fewer-claims-succeed-payouts-rise/.

5. "Medical Malpractice Statistics and Lawsuit Information," Weltchek, Mallahan and Weltchek, https://www.wmwlawfirm.com/facts-statistics-involving-medical-malpractice-law suits/, accessed February 14, 2018.

6. David H. Sohn, "Negligence, Genuine Error, and Litigation," *International Journal of General Medicine*, no. 6 (2013): 49–56, retrieved from https://www.ncbi.nlm.nih.gov/pmc/articles/PMC3576054/, doi:10.2147/IJGM.S24256.

7. The National Practitioner Data Bank is the US Department of Health and Human Services' online database of medical-malpractice payments; visit them online at https://www.npdb.hrsa.gov/.

8. Kevin B. O'Reilly, "1 in 3 Physicians Has Been Sued; by Age 55, 1 in 2 Hit with Suit," American Medical Association (website), January 26, 2018, https://www.ama-assn.org/practice-management/sustainability/1-3-physicians-has-been-sued-age-55-1-2-hit-suit.

9. Anna Almendrala, "Many Doctors Who Face Malpractice Suits Are Serial Offenders," *HuffPost Life*, January 29, 2016, https://www.huffpost.com/entry/doctors-malpractice-research_n_56a94bece4b05e4e37033d00.

10. David H. Sohn, "Negligence, Genuine Error, and Litigation," *International Journal of General Medicine*, no. 6 (2013): 49–56, retrieved from https://www.ncbi.nlm.nih.gov/pmc/articles/PMC3576054/, doi:10.2147/IJGM.S24256.

11. "Can We Predict Which Doctors Will Face Malpractice Suits?" Baker and Gilchrist (website), May 5, 2016, https://www.bakerandgilchrist.com/blog/predicting-doctors-will-face-malpractice-suits-look-complaints/.

12. David H. Sohn, "Negligence, Genuine Error, and Litigation," *International Journal of General Medicine*, no. 6 (2013): 49–56, retrieved from https://www.ncbi.nlm.nih.gov/pmc/articles/PMC3576054/, doi:10.2147/IJGM.S24256.

13. Ibid.

14. Michelle M. Mello, Amitabh Chandra, Atul A. Gawande, and David M. Studdert, "National Costs of the Medical Liability System," *Health Affairs* 29, no. 9 (2010): 1569–77, retrieved from https://www.ncbi.nlm.nih.gov/pmc/articles/PMC3048809/, doi:10.1377/hlth aff.2009.0807.

15. US Congress, Office of Technology Assessment, *Defensive Medicine and Medical Malpractice, OTA-H--602* (Washington, DC: US Government Printing Office, 1994), https://www.princeton.edu/~ota/disk1/1994/9405/9405.PDF.

16. David Klingman, A. Russell Localio, Jeremy Sugarman, Judith L. Wagner, Philip T. Polishuk, Leah Wolfe, and Jacqueline A. Corrigan, "Measuring Defensive Medicine Using Clinical Scenario Surveys," *Journal of Health Politics, Policy and Law* 21, no. 2 (1996): 185–217.

17. Heather Lyu, Tim Xu, Daniel Brotman, Brandan Mayer-Blackwell, Michol Cooper, Michael Daniel, Elizabeth C. Wick, Vikas Saini, Shannon Brownlee, and Martin A. Makary, "Overtreatment in the United States," I. K. Moise, ed. *PLoS One* 12, no. 9 (2017): e0181970, https://journals.plos.org/plosone/article?id=10.1371/journal.pone.0181970, doi:10.1371/journal.pone.0181970.

18. US Congress, Office of Technology Assessment, *Defensive Medicine and Medical Malpractice, OTA-H--602* (Washington, DC: US Government Printing Office, 1994), https://www.princeton.edu/~ota/disk1/1994/9405/9405.PDF.

19. Heather Lyu, Tim Xu, Daniel Brotman, Brandan Mayer-Blackwell, Michol Cooper, Michael Daniel, Elizabeth C. Wick, Vikas Saini, Shannon Brownlee, and Martin A. Makary,

"Overtreatment in the United States," Moise IK, ed. *PLoS One* 12, no. 9 (2017): e0181970, https://journals.plos.org/plosone/article?id=10.1371/journal.pone.0181970, doi:10.1371/journal.pone.0181970.

20. Anna Almendrala, "Many Doctors Who Face Malpractice Suits Are Serial Offenders," *HuffPost Life*, January 29, 2016, https://www.huffpost.com/entry/doctors-malpractice-research_n_56a94bece4b05e4e37033d00.

21. "A New Approach to Medical Malpractice," Leeseberg and Valentine (website), July 26, 2017, https://www.leesebergvalentine.com/blog/2017/07/a-new-approach-to-medical-mal practice.shtml.

22. "Communication and Optimal Resolution (CANDOR) Toolkit," Agency for Healthcare Research and Quality, last reviewed September 2017, https://www.ahrq.gov/professionals/quality-patient-safety/patient-safety-resources/resources/candor/introduction.html.

23. "A New Approach to Medical Malpractice," Leeseberg and Valentine (website), July 26, 2017, https://www.leesebergvalentine.com/blog/2017/07/a-new-approach-to-medical-mal practice.shtml.

24. Philip K. Howard and Rebecca G. Maine, "Health Courts May Be Best Cure for What Ails the Liability System," *Bulletin of the American College of Surgeons*, March 2, 2013, http://bulletin.facs.org/2013/03/health-courts-best-cure/.

25. "Can We Predict Which Doctors Will Face Malpractice Suits?" Baker and Gilchrist (website), May 5, 2016, https://www.bakerandgilchrist.com/blog/predicting-doctors-will-face-malpractice-suits-look-complaints/.

# 11. MYTH: IN THE UNITED STATES THERE IS A SAFETY NET OF GOVERNMENT HEALTH PROGRAMS FOR THE POOR

1. HealthCare.gov has posted the entirety of the Affordable Care Act (sometimes known as "Obamacare") online at https://www.healthcare.gov/where-can-i-read-the-affordable-care-act/.

2. Andrew P. Wilpur, Steffie Woolhandler, Karen E. Lasser, Danny McCormick, David H. Bor, and David U. Himmelstein, "Health Insurance and Mortality in US Adults," *American Journal of Public Health* 99, no. 12 (2009): 2289–95, retrieved from https://www.ncbi.nlm.nih.gov/pmc/articles/PMC2775760/, doi:10.2105/AJPH.2008.157685.

3. S. Craig Thomas, Robert A. Greevy, and Arthur Garson Jr., "Effect of Grand-Aides Nurse Extenders on Readmissions and Emergency Department Visits in Medicare Patients with Heart Failure," *American Journal of Cardiology* 121, no. 11 (2018): 1336–42, https://www.ajconline.org/article/S0002-9149(18)30248-0/pdf, doi:10.1016/j.amjcard.2018.02.012.

4. Christine D. Hsu, Xioyan Wang, David V. Habif Jr., Cynthia X. Ma, and Kimberly J. Johnson, "Breast Cancer Stage Variation and Survival in Association with Insurance Status and Sociodemographic Factors in US Women 18 to 64 Years Old," *Cancer* 123, no. 16 (2017): 3125–31, https://onlinelibrary.wiley.com/doi/full/10.1002/cncr.30722, doi:10.1002/cncr.30722.

5. Sarah Stark Casagrande and Catherine C. Cowie, "Health Insurance Coverage among People with and without Diabetes in the U.S. Adult Population," *Diabetes Care* 35, no. 11 (2012): 2243–49, http://care.diabetesjournals.org/content/35/11/2243, doi:10.2337/dc12-0257.

6. "How Health Insurance Impacts Prenatal Care," *Every Mother Counts*, August 19, 2014, https://blog.everymothercounts.org/how-health-insurance-impacts-prenatal-care-501c51c 03012.

7. "Health Insurance Coverage of the Total Population (Timeframe: 2014)," Henry J. Kaiser Family Foundation (website), https://www.kff.org/other/state-indicator/total-population/?dataView=1&currentTimeframe=3&sortModel=%7B"colId":"Location","sort":"asc"%7D, accessed February 13, 2018.

8. "Key Facts about the Uninsured Population," Henry J. Kaiser Family Foundation (website), December 7, 2018, https://www.kff.org/uninsured/fact-sheet/key-facts-about-the-uninsured-population/; "US States: Population and Ranking," *Enchanted Learning*, http://www.enchantedlearning.com/usa/states/population.shtml, accessed February 13, 2018.

9. S. Craig Thomas, Robert A. Greevy, and Arthur Garson Jr., "Effect of Grand-Aides Nurse Extenders on Readmissions and Emergency Department Visits in Medicare Patients with Heart Failure," *American Journal of Cardiology* 121, no. 11 (2018): 1336–42, https://www.ajconline.org/article/S0002-9149(18)30248-0/pdf, doi:10.1016/j.amjcard.2018.02.012.

10. Robin Rudowitz, Samantha Artiga, and Rachel Arguello, "Children's Health Coverage: Medicaid, CHIP and the ACA," Henry J. Kaiser Family Foundation (website), March 26, 2014, https://www.kff.org/health-reform/issue-brief/childrens-health-coverage-medicaid-chip-and-the-aca/.

11. Jessica C. Smith and Carla Medalia, "Health Insurance Coverage in the United States: 2013," United States Census Bureau, September 16, 2014, https://www.census.gov/library/publications/2014/demo/p60-250.html.

12. "TMC SURVEY 4-10-2015.pptx," retrieved from https://www.dropbox.com/s/4yf61fdsq9vt3n6/Houston%20Chronicle%2C%20April%2027%2C%202015.pdf?dl=0.

13. "Health Insurance Coverage of the Total Population (Timeframe: 2014)," Henry J. Kaiser Family Foundation (website), https://www.kff.org/other/state-indicator/total-population/?dataView=1&currentTimeframe=3&sortModel=%7B"colId":"Location","sort":"asc"%7D, accessed February 13, 2018.

14. Juliette Cubanski Tricia Neuman, Anthony Damico, and Karen Smith, "Medicare Beneficiaries' Out-of-Pocket Health Care Spending as a Share of Income Now and Projections for the Future—Report—9129," Henry J. Kaiser Family Foundation (website), January 26, 2018 https://www.kff.org/report-section/medicare-beneficiaries-out-of-pocket-health-care-spending-as-a-share-of-income-now-and-projections-for-the-future-report/.

15. "2013 Poverty Guidelines," Office of the Assistant Secretary for Planning and Evaluation, December 1, 2013, https://aspe.hhs.gov/2013-poverty-guidelines.

16. Carmen Denavas-Walt and Bernadette D. Proctor, "Income and Poverty in the United States: 2013," September 16, 2014, https://www.census.gov/library/publications/2014/demo/p60-249.html.

17. Robin Rudowitz, Samantha Artiga, and Rachel Arguello, "Children's Health Coverage: Medicaid, CHIP and the ACA," Henry J. Kaiser Family Foundation (website), March 26, 2014, https://www.kff.org/health-reform/issue-brief/childrens-health-coverage-medicaid-chip-and-the-aca/.

18. "The Children's Health Insurance Program," Georgetown University Health Policy Institute, Center for Children and Families (website), February 6, 2017, https://ccf.georgetown.edu/2017/02/06/about-chip/.

19. "CHIP Coverage for Pregnant Women," March of Dimes (website), May 2014, https://www.marchofdimes.org/materials/chip-coverage-for-pregnant-women-may-2014.pdf.

20. Monica Alba, "The VA by the Numbers: How Big Is It and Who Uses It?" NBC News, May 9, 2014, https://www.nbcnews.com/storyline/va-hospital-scandal/va-numbers-how-big-it-who-uses-it-n101771.

21. "Hospitals by Ownership Type (Timeframe: 2016)," Henry J. Kaiser Family Foundation (website), https://www.kff.org/other/state-indicator/hospitals-by-ownership/?dataView=1&cur

rentTimeframe=0&sortModel=%7B"colId":"Location","sort":"asc"%7D, accessed February 25, 2018.

22. Michelle Ko, Jack Needleman, Kathryn Pitkin Derose, Miriam J. Laugesen, and Ninez A. Ponce, "Residential Segregation and the Survival of U.S. Urban Public Hospitals," *Medical Care Research and Review* 71, no. 3 (2014): 243–60, doi:10.1177/1077558713515079.

23. "Federally Qualified Health Centers," Health Resources and Services Administration (website), last reviewed May 2018 https://www.hrsa.gov/opa/eligibility-and-registration/health-centers/fqhc/index.html.

24. Elaine J. Heisler, "Federal Health Centers: An Overview," Congressional Research Service, May 17, 2017, https://fas.org/sgp/crs/misc/R43937.pdf.

25. Catherine Hoffman and Susan Starr Sered, "Threadbare: Holes in America's Health Care Safety Net," Kaiser Commission on Medicaid and the Uninsured, November 2005, https://kaiserfamilyfoundation.files.wordpress.com/2013/01/threadbare-holes-in-america-s-health-care-safety-net-report.pdf.

26. Candice L. Williams, William O. Cooper, Leanne S. Balmer, Judith A. Dudley, Patricia S. Gideon, Michelle M. DeRanieri, Shannon M. Stratton, and S. Todd Callahan, "Evaluation and Disposition of Medicaid-Insured Children and Adolescents with Suicide Attempts," *Academic Pediatrics* 15, no. 1 (2015): 36–40, doi:10.1016/j.acap.2014.04.005.

27. "Medicaid-to-Medicare Fee Index (Timeframe: 2016)," Henry J. Kaiser Family Foundation (website), https://www.kff.org/medicaid/state-indicator/medicaid-to-medicare-fee-index/?currentTimeframe=0&sortModel=%7B"colId":"Location","sort":"asc"%7D, accessed November 1, 2018; Daria Pelech, "An Analysis of Private-Sector Prices for Physician Services," Congressional Budget Office, June 26, 2017, https://www.cbo.gov/system/files/115th-congress-2017-2018/presentation/52818-dp-presentation.pdf.

28. Sandra L. Decker, "In 2011 Nearly One-Third of Physicians Said They Would Not Accept New Medicaid Patients, but Rising Fees May Help," *Health Affairs* 31, no. 8 (2012): 1673–79, https://www.healthaffairs.org/doi/full/10.1377/hlthaff.2012.0294, doi:10.1377/hlthaff.2012.0294.

29. "Armstrong v. Exceptional Child Center, Inc.," Constitutional Accountability Center (website), https://www.theusconstitution.org/litigation/armstrong-v-exceptional-child-center-inc-u-s-sup-ct/, accessed November 1, 2018.

30. S. Craig Thomas, Robert A. Greevy, and Arthur Garson Jr., "Effect of Grand-Aides Nurse Extenders on Readmissions and Emergency Department Visits in Medicare Patients with Heart Failure," *American Journal of Cardiology* 121, no. 11 (2018): 1336–42, https://www.ajconline.org/article/S0002-9149(18)30248-0/pdf, doi:10.1016/j.amjcard.2018.02.012.

31. John Holahan, Matthew Buettgens, Caitlin Carroll, and Stan Dorn, "The Cost and Coverage Implications of the ACA Medicaid Expansion: National and State-by-State Analysis; Executive Summary," Kaiser Commission on Medicaid and the Uninsured, November 2012, https://kaiserfamilyfoundation.files.wordpress.com/2013/01/8384_es.pdf.

32. *National Federation of Independent Business et al. v. Sebelius, Secretary of Health and Human Services, et al.*, 393 U.S. (2012), https://www.supremecourt.gov/opinions/11pdf/11-393c3a2.pdf.

33. "Status of State Action on the Medicaid Expansion Decision (Timeframe: as of February 13, 2019)," Henry J. Kaiser Family Foundation (website), https://www.kff.org/health-reform/state-indicator/state-activity-around-expanding-medicaid-under-the-affordable-care-act/.

34. Alan M. Preston, "Why Expanding Medicaid Is a Bad Idea for Texas," *San Antonio Express-News*, September 24, 2016, https://www.mysanantonio.com/opinion/commentary/article/Why-expanding-Medicaid-is-a-bad-idea-for-Texas-9242918.php.

35. "Part I. Medicaid and CHIP: An Overview; Chapter 1: Medicaid and CHIP Basics," in *Texas Medicaid and CHIP in Perspective*, 11th edition, 1–16 (Austin: Texas Health and Human Services Commission, 2017), https://hhs.texas.gov/sites/default/files/documents/laws-regulations/reports-presentations/2017/medicaid-chip-perspective-11th-edition/11th-edition-chapter1.pdf.

36. "Updated Estimates of the Effects of the Insurance Coverage Provisions of the Affordable Care Act, April 2014," Congressional Budget Office, April 2014, http://www.cbo.gov/sites/default/files/cbofiles/attachments/45231-ACA_Estimates.pdf.

37. "Focus on Health Reform: Summary of the Affordable Care Act," Henry J. Kaiser Family Foundation (website), 2013, http://files.kff.org/attachment/fact-sheet-summary-of-the-affordable-care-act.

38. Hubert Humphrey, remarks at the dedication of the Hubert H. Humphrey Building, November 1, 1977, *Congressional Record*, November 4, 1977, vol. 123, p. 37287. See also Don Berwick, "Healthcare, Technology and Government 2.0: The Moral Test," December 11, 2011, https://www.coloradoafp.org/wp-content/uploads/2017/01/Berwick-The-Moral-Test-12-2011.pdf.

39. Zac Auter, "U.S. Uninsured Rate Rises to 11.7%," Gallup, July 10, 2017, https://news.gallup.com/poll/213665/uninsured-rate-rises.aspx.

# 12. MYTH: PEOPLE WHO WORK CAN AFFORD HEALTH INSURANCE

1. Esther Bloom, "Kellyanne Conway: Those on Medicaid Who Will Lose Insurance Can Get Jobs," CNBC, June 25, 2017, https://www.cnbc.com/2017/06/25/kellyanne-conway-those-on-medicaid-who-will-lose-insurance-can-get-jobs.html.

2. "Percent of Private Sector Establishments That Offer Health Insurance to Employees (Timeframe: 2017)," Henry J. Kaiser Family Foundation (website), https://www.kff.org/other/state-indicator/percent-of-firms-offering-coverage/, accessed November 3, 2018.

3. "Key Facts about the Uninsured Population," Henry J. Kaiser Family Foundation (website), December 7, 2018, https://www.kff.org/uninsured/fact-sheet/key-facts-about-the-uninsured-population/.

4. "Health Insurance Coverage of the Total Population (Timeframe: 2017)," Henry J. Kaiser Family Foundation (website), https://www.kff.org/other/state-indicator/total-population/, accessed February 12, 2018.

5. "Employee Retirement Income Security Act (ERISA)," United States Department of Labor, https://www.dol.gov/general/topic/retirement/erisa, accessed February 12, 2018.

6. Figure 10.1, "Percentage of Covered Workers Enrolled in a Self-Funded Plan, by Firm Size, 2017," in "2017 Employer Health Benefits Survey; Section 10: Plan Funding," Henry J. Kaiser Family Foundation (website), https://www.kff.org/report-section/ehbs-2017-section-10-plan-funding/figure101, accessed February 12, 2018.

7. "Health Insurance Coverage of the Total Population (Timeframe: 2017)," Henry J. Kaiser Family Foundation (website), https://www.kff.org/other/state-indicator/total-population/, accessed February 12, 2018.

8. Jenny Deam, "Health Care Survey Yields Surprises for the Medical Community," *Houston Chronicle*, April 27, 2015, https://www.houstonchronicle.com/business/medical/article/Health-care-survey-yields-surprises-for-the-6227381.php.

9. Joseph Antos, "End the Exemption for Employer-Provided Health Care," *New York Times*, updated December 6, 2016, https://www.nytimes.com/roomfordebate/2015/04/14/the-worst-tax-breaks/end-the-exemption-for-employer-provided-health-care.

10. "Tax Policy Center's Briefing Book: Q: How Does the Tax Exclusion for Employer-Sponsored Health Insurance Work?" Tax Policy Center (website), http://www.taxpolicycenter.org/briefing-book/how-does-tax-exclusion-employer-sponsored-health-insurance-work, accessed February 12, 2018.

11. "Economic News Release: Employer Costs for Employee Compensation News Release Text," Bureau of Labor Statistics (website), December 14, 2018, https://www.bls.gov/news.release/ecec.nr0.htm.

12. Visit the Leapfrog Group online at http://www.leapfroggroup.org/.

13. Austin Ramzy, "McCain's Vote Provides Dramatic Moment in 7-Year Battle Over Obamacare," *New York Times*, July 28, 2017, https://www.nytimes.com/2017/07/28/us/politics/john-mccain-vote-trump-obamacare.html.

14. Christina Merhar, "FAQ—How Many Small Businesses Offer Health Insurance?" PeopleKeep (website), February 5, 2015, https://www.peoplekeep.com/blog/faq-how-many-small-businesses-offer-health-insurance.

15. Ibid.

16. Austin Ramzy, "McCain's Vote Provides Dramatic Moment in 7-Year Battle Over Obamacare," *New York Times*, July 28, 2017, https://www.nytimes.com/2017/07/28/us/politics/john-mccain-vote-trump-obamacare.html.

17. "Small and Large Business Health Insurance: State and Federal Roles," National Conference of State Legislatures, updated September 12, 2018, http://www.ncsl.org/research/health/small-business-health-insurance.aspx.

18. "Health Insurance Coverage of the Total Population (Timeframe: 2017)," Henry J. Kaiser Family Foundation (website), https://www.kff.org/other/state-indicator/total-population/, accessed February 12, 2018.

19. "Average Individual Health Insurance Premiums Increased 99% since 2013, the Year before Obamacare, & Family Premiums Increased 140%, According to eHealth.com Shopping Data," eHealth Insurance, January 23, 2017, https://news.ehealthinsurance.com/news/average-individual-health-insurance-premiums-increased-99-since-2013-the-year-before-obamacare-family-premiums-increased-140-according-to-ehealth-com-shopping-data.

20. "2013 Poverty Guidelines," Office of the Assistant Secretary for Planning and Evaluation, December 1, 2013, https://aspe.hhs.gov/2013-poverty-guidelines; Alexa Mason, "Can You Make It on a $30,000 Budget?" *Cult of Money*, July 1, 2015, http://www.cultofmoney.com/2015/07/01/can-you-make-it-on-a-30000-budget/; "Think You Couldn't Live on $30,000 a Year? Yes, You Can!" National Debt Relief (website), November 20, 2013, https://www.nationaldebtrelief.com/think-couldnt-live-30000-year-yes-can/; "How to Budget Living on $30000 a Year," *My Unentitled Life*, July 2014, http://www.myunentitledlife.com/2014/07/budget-living-30000-year.html.

21. "31 Million People Were Underinsured in 2014; Many Skipped Needed Health Care and Depleted Savings to Pay Medical Bills," Commonwealth Fund (website), May 20, 2015, http://www.commonwealthfund.org/publications/press-releases/2015/may/underinsurance-brief-release.

22. Arthur "Tim" Garson, Stephen H. Linder, and Ryan Holeywell, "The Nation's Pulse: The Texas Medical Center's Customer & Physician Survey," slides of survey findings, Texas Medical Center, 2017, https://www.tmc.edu/health-policy/wp-content/uploads/sites/5/2017/09/2017NationsPulsePresentation.pdf.

23. Joseph Antos, "End the Exemption for Employer-Provided Health Care," *New York Times*, updated December 6, 2016, https://www.nytimes.com/roomfordebate/2015/04/14/the-worst-tax-breaks/end-the-exemption-for-employer-provided-health-care.

24. Ibid.

25. Arthur "Tim" Garson Jr., "Half of U.S. Can't Afford Health Care. Doctor Salaries Could Cut Costs," *USA Today*, October 23, 2017, https://www.usatoday.com/story/opinion/2017/10/23/cut-health-costs-put-doctors-on-salaries-arthur-tim-garson-jr-column/777179001/; "How to Make the Affordable Care Act Affordable," *HuffPost*, November 3, 2017, https://www.huffingtonpost.com/arthur-tim-garson-jr-md-mph-macc-/how-to-make-the-affordabl_b_1277 9180.html.

26. "Summary of the Affordable Care Act," Henry J. Kaiser Family Foundation (website), March 2017, http://files.kff.org/attachment/Summary-of-the-Affordable-Care-Act.

27. "Hazardous Health Plans: Coverage Gaps Can Leave You in Big Trouble," *Consumer Reports*, last updated May 2009, https://www.consumerreports.org/cro/2012/05/hazardous-health-plans/index.htm.

28. Arthur "Tim" Garson Jr., "One of Many Problems with Short-Term Insurance Plans: Consumers Can't Understand Them," March 6, 2018, https://www.statnews.com/2018/03/06/short-term-health-insurance-consumers/.

29. Stephen Miller, "What Individual Mandate Repeal Means for Employers," Society for Human Resource Management (website), December 22, 2017, https://www.shrm.org/resourcesandtools/hr-topics/benefits/pages/individual-mandate-repeal-affects-employers.aspx.

30. Graph, "Cumulative Increases in Health Insurance Premiums, Workers' Contributions to Premiums, Inflation, and Workers' Earnings, 1992–2012," in "Employer-Sponsored Health Coverage: Release Slides," Henry J. Kaiser Family Foundation (website), September 11, 2012, https://kaiserfamilyfoundation.files.wordpress.com/2013/04/2012-employer-health-benefits-chart-pack-private-insurance-091112.pdf; "Figure B, Average Annual Health Insurance Premiums and Worker Contributions for Family Coverage, 2007–2017," in "2017 Employer Health Benefits Survey," Henry J. Kaiser Family Foundation (website), September 19, 2017, https://www.kff.org/report-section/ehbs-2017-summary-of-findings/figureb.

31. "How Much Does Obamacare Cost in 2017?" eHealth, https://resources.ehealthinsurance.com/affordable-care-act/much-obamacare-cost-2017, accessed March 15, 2018.

32. "The Uninsured Rate among Nonelderly Adults, 2008–2017," figure, Henry J. Kaiser Family Foundation (website), https://www.kff.org/uninsured/, accessed November 3, 2018.

## 13. MYTH: THE UNINSURED GET ADEQUATE CARE IN THE EMERGENCY DEPARTMENT

1. J. Goodrich, "Let Them Go to Emergency Rooms," *The American Prospect*, July 12, 2007, http://prospect.org/article/let-them-go-emergency-rooms.

2. Diane J. Angelini and Laura R. Mahlmeister, "Liability and Triage: Management of EMTALA Regulations and Common Obstetric Risks," *Journal of Midwifery and Women's Health* 50, no. 6 (2005): 472–78, doi.org/10.1016/j.jmwh.2005.07.006.

3. David Doyle, "Emergency Rooms Continue to Serve as Patients' Primary-Care Provider," *Physicians Practice* (blog), March 8, 2013, http://www.physicianspractice.com/blog/emergency-rooms-continue-serve-patients-primary-care-provider.

4. Ruohua Annetta Zhou, Katherine Baicker, Sarah Taubman, and Amy N. Finkelstein, "The Uninsured Do Not Use the Emergency Department More—They Use Other Care Less," *Health Affairs* 36, no. 12 (2017): 2115–22, doi:10.1377/hlthaff.2017.0218.

5. "Study: 71% of ED Visits Unnecessary, Avoidable," *Becker's Hospital Review*, April 25, 2013, https://www.beckershospitalreview.com/patient-flow/study-71-of-ed-visits-unneces sary-avoidable.html.

6. Wojciech Pisarek, Jean-Claude Auwera, Mike Smet, Pierre Damme, and Jan Stroobants, "Insured versus Uninsured Patients in the Emergency Room: Is There a Difference?" *European Journal of Emergency Medicine* 10, no. 4 (2003): 314–17, doi:10.1097/01.mej.0000104 024.33339.47.

7. Benjamin C. Sun, Renee Y. Hsia, Robert E. Weiss, David Zingmond, Li-Jung Liang, Weijuan Han, Heather McCreath, and Steven M. Asch, "Effect of Emergency Department Crowding on Outcomes of Admitted Patients," *Annals of Emergency Medicine* 61, no. 6 (2013): 605–11.e6, doi:10.1016/j.annemergmed.2012.10.026.

8. Jesse M. Pines and Zachary F. Meisel, "The Diverted Ambulance: How ER Crowding Kills," *Time*, January 27, 2011, http://content.time.com/time/health/article/0,8599,2079935,00. html, doi:10.1111/j.1553-2712.2008.00295.x.

9. Institute of Medicine, *Hospital-Based Emergency Care: At the Breaking Point* (Washington, DC: National Academies Press, 2007); Andrew P. Wilper, Steffie Woolhandler, Karen E. Lasser, Danny McCormick, David H. Bor, and David U. Himmelstein, "Health Insurance and Mortality in US Adults," *American Journal of Public Health* 99, no. 12 (2009): 2289–95, https://www.ncbi.nlm.nih.gov/pmc/articles/PMC2775760/, doi:10.2105/AJP.2008.157685.

10. Ruohua Annetta Zhou, Katherine Baicker, Sarah Taubman, and Amy N. Finkelstein, "The Uninsured Do Not Use the Emergency Department More—They Use Other Care Less," *Health Affairs* 36, no. 12 (2017): 2115–22, doi:10.1377/hlthaff.2017.0218.

11. Christine D. Hsu, Xioyan Wang, David V. Habif Jr., Cynthia X. Ma, and Kimberly J. Johnson, "Breast Cancer Stage Variation and Survival in Association with Insurance Status and Sociodemographic Factors in US Women 18 to 64 Years Old," *Cancer* 123, no. 16 (2017): 3125–31, https://onlinelibrary.wiley.com/doi/full/10.1002/cncr.30722, doi:10.1002/cncr .30722.

12. Andrew P. Wilper, Steffie Woolhandler, Karen E. Lasser, Danny McCormick, David H. Bor, and David U. Himmelstein, "Health Insurance and Mortality in US Adults," *American Journal of Public Health* 99, no. 12 (2009): 2289–95, https://www.ncbi.nlm.nih.gov/pmc/ articles/PMC2775760/, doi:10.2105/AJP.2008.157685.

13. "How Health Insurance Impacts Prenatal Care," Every Mother Counts (website), August 19, 2014, https://blog.everymothercounts.org/how-health-insurance-impacts-prenatal-care-501c51c03012.

14. "The Uninsured: Access to Medical Care Fact Sheet," American College of Emergency Physicians, last updated 2016, http://newsroom.acep.org/2009-01-04-the-uninsured-access-to-medical-care-fact-sheet.

15. Lorena Lopez-Gonzalez, Gary T. Pickens, Raynard Washington, and Audrey J. Weiss, "Characteristics of Medicaid and Uninsured Hospitalizations, 2012," Health Care Cost and Utilization Project statistical brief 182, Agency for Healthcare Research and Quality, October 2014, https://www.hcup-us.ahrq.gov/reports/statbriefs/sb182-Medicaid-Uninsured-Hospitaliza tions-2012.pdf.

16. Healthcare Cost and Utilization Project, "Overview Statistics for Inpatient Hospital Stays," in *HCUP Facts and Figures: Statistics on Hospital-Based Care in the United States, 2009* (Rockville, MD: Agency for Healthcare Research and Quality, 2011), https://www.ncbi. nlm.nih.gov/books/NBK91986/.

17. Maya Bunik, Judith E. Glazner, Vijayalaxmi Chandramouli, Caroline Bublitz Emsermann, Teresa Hegarty, and Allison Kempe, "Pediatric Telephone Call Centers: How Do They Affect Health Care Use and Costs?" *Pediatrics* 119, no. 2 (2007): e305–13, doi:10.1542/peds.2006-1511.

18. Arthur Garson, Donna M. Green, Lia Rodriguez, Richard Beech, and Christopher Nye, "A New Corps of Trained Grand-Aides Has the Potential to Extend Reach of Primary Care Workforce and Save Money," *Health Affairs* 31, no. 5 (2012): 1016–21, https://www.healthaffairs.org/doi/full/10.1377/hlthaff.2011.0859, doi:10.1377/hlthaff.2011.0859.

19. Arthur "Tim" Garson Jr., "Patients Need to Know What a True Emergency Is before Going to the ER," *TribTalk*, August 20, 2018, https://www.tribtalk.org/2018/08/20/patients-need-to-know-what-a-true-emergency-is-before-going-to-the-er/.

20. Amanda Moore, "Tracking Down Martin Luther King, Jr.'s Words on Health Care," *Huffing Post*, updated March 20, 2013, https://www.huffingtonpost.com/amanda-moore/martin-luther-king-health-care_b_2506393.html.

# 14. MYTH: THE MARKET CAN FIX HEALTH CARE

1. Tom Coburn, "Get Government Out and Let Markets Work in Health Care," *Hill*, November 23, 2017, http://thehill.com/opinion/healthcare/361695-get-government-out-and-let-markets-work-in-health-care; Ken Blackwell, "Let the Market Fix Health Care," *Daily Caller*, February 20, 2017, https://dailycaller.com/2017/02/20/let-the-market-fix-health-care/.

2. Sandra Schickele, "The Economic Case for Public Subsidy of the Internet," working paper, Sonoma State University, April 6, 1993, text retrieved from https://totseans.com/totse/en/politics/economic_documents/schickel.html.

3. Robert Pear, "Why Your Pharmacist Can't Tell You That $20 Prescription Could Cost Only $8," *New York Times*, February 24, 2018, https://www.nytimes.com/2018/02/24/us/politics/pharmacy-benefit-managers-gag-clauses.html.

4. Dave Schuler, "Is Healthcare a Luxury Good?" *The Glittering Eye*, August 9, 2009, http://theglitteringeye.com/is-healthcare-a-luxury-good/.

5. "Definition of 'Moral Hazard,'" *Economic Times*, https://economictimes.indiatimes.com/definition/moral-hazard, accessed February 9, 2018.

6. Shankar Vedantam, "Money May Be Motivating Doctors to Do More C-Sections," *Hidden Brain*, NPR, August 30, 2013, https://www.npr.org/sections/health-shots/2013/08/30/216479305/money-may-be-motivating-doctors-to-do-more-c-sections.

7. Katherine J. Aikin, John L. Swasy, and Amie C. Braman, "Patient and Physician Attitudes and Behaviors Associated with DTC Promotion of Prescription Drugs: Summary of FDA Survey Research Results; Final Report," November 19, 2004, https://www.fda.gov/downloads/AboutFDA/CentersOffices/OfficeofMedicalProductsandTobacco/CDER/UCM600276.pdf.

8. Tom Leys, "Iowa Teen's $1 Million-per-Month Illness Is No Longer a Secret," *Des Moines Register*, May 31, 2017, https://www.desmoinesregister.com/story/news/health/2017/05/31/hemophilia-patient-costing-iowa-insurer-1-million-per-month/356179001/.

9. Terrence P. Jeffrey, "Census Bureau: 118,395,000 on 'Government Health Insurance' in 2015; 28,966,000 Uninsured for Entire Year," CNSNews.com, September 13, 2016, https://www.cnsnews.com/news/article/terence-p-jeffrey/census-bureau-118395000-government-health-insurance-2015-28966000.

10. Arthur "Tim" Garson, Stephen H. Linder, and Ryan Holeywell, "The Nation's Pulse: The Texas Medical Center's Customer & Physician Survey," slides of survey findings, Texas Medical Center, 2017, https://www.tmc.edu/health-policy/wp-content/uploads/sites/5/2017/09/2017NationsPulsePresentation.pdf.

11. Atul Gawande, "Health Care's Price Conundrum," *The New Yorker*, December 18, 2015, https://www.newyorker.com/news/news-desk/health-cares-cost-conundrum-squared.

12. Luisa Franzini, Osama I. Mikhail, and Jonathan S. Skinner, "McAllen And El Paso Revisited: Medicare Variations Not Always Reflected in the Under-Sixty-Five Population," *Health Affairs* 29, no. 12 (2010): 2302–9, https://www.healthaffairs.org/doi/pdf/10.1377/hlthaff.2010.0492, doi:10.1377/hlthaff.2010.0492.

13. Adam Cancryn and Louis Nelson, "Trump Says Health Care Executive Order Will Allow Coverage to Be Sold across State Lines," Politico, October 10, 2017, https://www.politico.com/story/2017/10/10/trump-executive-order-health-care-243622.

14. Michael E. Porter and Elizabeth Teisberg, "Redefining Competition in Health Care," *Harvard Business Review*, June 2004, https://hbr.org/2004/06/redefining-competition-in-health-care.

15. "Insurance Commissioner's Plain Language Campaign: Keep It Simple," Texas Department of Insurance (website), May 23, 2018, https://www.tdi.texas.gov/news/2018/tdi05232018.html.

16. Cory Franklin, "The Bond between Patient and Physician Is in Jeopardy," *Chicago Tribune*, December 31, 2014, http://www.chicagotribune.com/news/opinion/commentary/ct-physician-patient-bond-jeopardy-perspec-0101-20141231-story.html.

17. In the interests of full disclosure, Garson is an elected member of the National Academy of Medicine.

18. Julie P. Phillips, Stephen M. Petterson, Andrew W. Bazemore, and Robert L. Phillips, "A Retrospective Analysis of the Relationship between Medical Student Debt and Primary Care Practice in the United States," *Annals of Family Medicine* 12, no. 6 (2014): 542–49, http://www.annfammed.org/content/12/6/542.long, doi:10.1370/afm.1697.

19. Lisa Rhodes, "Student Loan Forgiveness (And Other Ways the Government Can Help You Repay Your Loans)," *Homeroom* (blog), October 8, 2014, https://blog.ed.gov/2014/10/student-loan-forgiveness-and-other-ways-the-government-can-help-you-repay-your-loans-2/.

## 15. MYTH: DOCTORS AND HOSPITALS SHOULD BE PAID SEPARATELY FOR EACH SERVICE THEY PERFORM

1. Michael W. Rich and Kenneth E. Freedland, "Effect of DRGs on Three-Month Readmission Rate of Geriatric Patients with Congestive Heart Failure," *American Journal of Public Health* 78, no. 6 (1988): 680–82, http://ajph.aphapublications.org/doi/pdf/10.2105/AJPH.78.6.680.

2. Lauren A. McCormack and Russel T. Burge, "Diffusion of Medicare's RBRVS and Related Physician Payment Policies," *Health Care Financing Review* 16, no. 2 (1994): 159–73, https://www.ncbi.nlm.nih.gov/pmc/articles/PMC4193488/.

3. "Physician Fee Schedule," *CMS.gov*, last modified March 8, 2019, https://www.cms.gov/Medicare/Medicare-Fee-for-Service-Payment/PhysicianFeeSched/.

4. Nguyen Xuan Nguyen and Frederick William Derrick, "Physician Behavioral Response to a Medicare Price Reduction," *HSR: Health Services Research* 32, no. 3 (1997): 283–98, https://www.ncbi.nlm.nih.gov/pmc/articles/PMC1070191/pdf/hsresearch00035-0034.pdf.

5. Marcia Angell, "The Doctor as Double Agent," *Kennedy Institute of Ethics Journal* 3, no. 3 (1993): 279–86, doi:10.1353/ken.0.0253.

6. Ken Terry, "Do Doctors Give HMO Patients a Fair Shake?" *Medical Economics*, February 21, 2000, https://www.medicaleconomics.com/article/do-doctors-give-hmo-patients-fair-shake.

7. Milt Freudenheim, "H.M.O.'s Cope with a Backlash on Cost Cutting," *New York Times*, May 19, 1996, http://www.nytimes.com/1996/05/19/us/hmo-s-cope-with-a-backlash-on-cost-cutting.html.

8. M. Kim Marvel, Ronald M. Epstein, Kristine Flowers, and Howard B. Beckman, "Soliciting the Patient's Agenda: Have We Improved?" *Journal of the American Medical Association* 281, no. 3 (1999): 283–87, http://www.ncbi.nlm.nih.gov/pubmed/9918487, doi:10.1001/jama.281.3.283.

9. Donald M. Berwick and Andrew D. Hackbarth, "Eliminating Waste in US Health Care," *Journal of the American Medical Association* 307, no. 14 (2012): 1513–16, doi:10.1001/jama.2012.362.

10. Steven A. Schroeder and William Frist, "Phasing Out Fee-for-Service Payment," *New England Journal of Medicine* 368, no. 21 (2013): 2029–32, doi:10.1056/NEJMsb1302322.

11. Heather Lyu, Tim Xu, Daniel Brotman, Brandan Mayer-Blackwell, Michol Cooper, Michael Daniel, Elizabeth C. Wick, Vikas Saini, Shannon Brownlee, and Martin A. Makary, "Overtreatment in the United States," Moise IK, ed. *PLoS One* 12, no. 9 (2017): e0181970, https://journals.plos.org/plosone/article?id=10.1371/journal.pone.0181970, doi:10.1371/journal.pone.0181970.

12. Sylvia M. Burwell "Setting Value-Based Payment Goals—HHS Efforts to Improve U.S. Health Care," *New England Journal of Medicine* 372, no. 10 (2015): 897–99, doi:10.1056/NEJMp1500445.

13. Ryan Holeywell, "Is It Time to Start Paying Doctors Salaries?" *TMC News*, October 3 2017, http://www.tmc.edu/news/2017/10/time-start-paying-doctors-salaries/.

14. T. Gosden, F. Forland, I. S. Kristiansen, M. Sutton, B. Leese, A. Giuffrida, M. Sergison, and L Pedersen, "Capitation, Salary, Fee-for-Service and Mixed Systems of Payment: Effects on the Behaviour of Primary Care Physicians," *Cochrane Database Systematic Reviews*, no. 3 (2000), CD002215, doi:10.1002/14651858.CD002215.

# 16. MYTH: THE UNITED STATES WILL
# NEVER BE ABLE TO REDUCE THE COST OF MEDICAL CARE

1. Peter Wehrwein, "Value = (Quality + Outcomes) / Cost," *Managed Care Magazine*, August 16 2015, https://www.managedcaremag.com/archives/2015/8/value-quality-outcomes-cost.

2. Donald M. Berwick and Andrew D. Hackbarth, "Eliminating Waste in US Health Care," *Journal of the American Medical Association* 307, no. 14 (2012): 1513, doi:10.1001/jama.2012.362.

3. "EHR Adoption Rates and Statistics: 2012–2017," Practice Fusion (website), March 1, 2017, https://www.practicefusion.com/blog/ehr-adoption-rates/; "AMA Survey: Physician

Satisfaction with EHR Systems Has Plummeted," daily briefing, Advisory Board (website), August 13, 2015, https://www.advisory.com/daily-briefing/2015/08/13/ama-survey-physician-satisfaction-with-ehr-systems-has-plummeted.

4. Alfred Ng, "IBM's Watson Gives Proper Diagnosis after Doctors Were Stumped," *New York Daily News*, August 7, 2016, http://www.nydailynews.com/news/world/ibm-watson-proper-diagnosis-doctors-stumped-article-1.2741857.

5. T. Gosden, L. Pedersen, and D. Torgerson, "How Should We Pay Doctors? A Systematic Review of Salary Payments and Their Effect on Doctor Behaviour," *QJM* 92, no. 1 (1999): 47–55, https://academic.oup.com/qjmed/article/92/1/47/1550410, doi:10.1093/qjmed/92.1.47.

6. Hope Kenefick, Jason Lee, and Valerie Fleishman, "Improving Physician Adherence to Clinical Practice Guidelines: Barriers and Strategies for Change," New England Healthcare Institute, February 2008, https://www.nehi.net/writable/publication_files/file/cpg_report_final.pdf.

7. "Advancing the *Choosing Wisely* Campaign in Clinical Practices and Communities," Choosing Wisely (website), October 2014, http://www.choosingwisely.org/wp-content/uploads/2014/10/Choosing-Wisely-Grant-Report.pdf.

8. Timothy K. Mackey and Bryan A. Liang, "The Role of Practice Guidelines in Medical Malpractice Litigation," *Virtual Mentor* 13, no. 1 (2011): 36–41, retrieved from https://journalofethics.ama-assn.org/article/role-practice-guidelines-medical-malpractice-litigation/2011-01, doi:10.1001/virtualmentor.2011.13.1.hlaw1-1101.

9. Melissa D. Aldridge and Amy S. Kelley, "The Myth regarding the High Cost of End-of-Life Care," *American Journal of Public Health* 105, no. 12 (2015): 2411–15, https://ajph.aphapublications.org/doi/pdf/10.2105/AJPH.2015.302889.

10. Don Gonyea, "How False Claims of Obamacare 'Death Panels' Stuck with the President," NPR, January 10, 2017, https://www.npr.org/2017/01/10/509164679/from-the-start-obama-struggled-with-fallout-from-a-kind-of-fake-news.

11. Mayo Clinic staff, "Living Wills and Advance Directives for Medical Decisions," Mayo Clinic (website), December 15, 2018, https://www.mayoclinic.org/healthy-lifestyle/consumer-health/in-depth/living-wills/art-20046303.

12. Elizabeth Newcomb, "Tom Petty and Your End-of-Life Wishes," *Next Avenue*, October 24, 2017, https://www.nextavenue.org/tom-petty-end-of-life-wishes/.

13. Ibid.

14. Lauren Hersch Nicholas, Kenneth M. Langa, Theodore J. Iwashyna, and David R. Weir, "Regional Variation in the Association between Advance Directives and End-of-Life Medicare Expenditures," *Journal of the American Medical Association* 306 (2011): 1447–53, https://jamanetwork.com/journals/jama/fullarticle/1104465.

15. David C. Goodman, Elliott S. Fisher, Chiang-hua Chang, Nancy E. Morden, Joseph O. Jacobson, Kimberly Murray, and Susan Miesfeldt, Kristen K. Bronner, ed., "Quality of End-of-Life Cancer Care for Medicare Beneficiaries: Regional and Hospital-Specific Analyses," Report of the Dartmouth Atlas Project, Dartmouth Institute for Health Policy and Clinical Practice, November 16, 2010, http://archive.dartmouthatlas.org/downloads/reports/Cancer_report_11_16_10.pdf.

16. "Palliative Care Information Act," New York State Department of Health (website), revised February 2011, https://www.health.ny.gov/professionals/patients/patient_rights/palliative_care/information_act.htm.

17. Adrienne L. Jones, Abigail J. Moss, and Lauren D. Harris-Kojetin, "Use of Advance Directives in Long-Term Care Populations," *NCHS Data Brief*, no. 54 (2011): 1–8, https://www.cdc.gov/nchs/data/databriefs/db54.pdf.

18. Lawrence S. Wissow, Amy Belote, Wade Kramer, Amy Compton-Phillips, Robert Kritzler, and Janathan P. Weiner, "Promoting Advance Directives among Elderly Primary Care Patients," *Journal of General Internal Medicine* 19, no. 9 (2004): 944–51, retrieved from https://www.ncbi.nlm.nih.gov/pmc/articles/PMC1492518/.

19. Jordan Rau, "Few Consumers Are Using Quality, Price Information to Make Health Decisions," Kaiser Health News, April 21, 2015, https://khn.org/news/few-consumers-are-using-quality-price-information-to-make-health-care-decisions/.

20. Susan T. Stewart, David M. Cutler, and Allison B. Rosen, "Forecasting the Effects of Obesity and Smoking on U.S. Life Expectancy," *New England Journal of Medicine* 361 (2009): 2252–60, https://www.nejm.org/doi/full/10.1056/NEJMsa0900459.

21. Arthur "Tim" Garson, Stephen H. Linder, and Ryan Holeywell, "The Nation's Pulse: The Texas Medical Center's Customer & Physician Survey," slides of survey findings, Texas Medical Center, 2017, https://www.tmc.edu/health-policy/wp-content/uploads/sites/5/2017/09/2017NationsPulsePresentation.pdf.

22. Arthur "Tim" Garson, Stephen H. Linder, and Ryan Holeywell, "The Nation's Pulse: The Texas Medical Center's Customer Survey," slides of survey findings, Texas Medical Center, 2018, https://www.tmc.edu/health-policy/wp-content/uploads/sites/5/2018/08/08_31_FINAL-US-SLIDES.pdf.

23. "More than Half of Consumers Now Buy on Their Beliefs," Edelman (website), June 8, 2017, https://www.edelman.com/news-awards/consumers-now-buy-on-beliefs-2017-earned-brand.

24. J. Michael McGinnis, Pamela Williams-Russo, and James R. Knickman, "The Case for More Active Policy Attention to Health Promotion," *Health Affairs* 21 (2002): 78–93, https://www.healthaffairs.org/doi/10.1377/hlthaff.21.2.78.

25. Marie T. Brown and Jennifer K. Bussell, "Medication Adherence: WHO Cares?" *Mayo Clinic Proceedings* 86, no. 4 (2011): 304–14, retrieved from https://www.ncbi.nlm.nih.gov/pmc/articles/PMC3068890/.

26. M. Christopher Roebuck, Joshua N. Liberman, Marin Gemmill-Toyama, and Troyen A. Brennan, "Medication Adherence Leads to Lower Health Care Use and Costs Despite Increased Drug Spending," *Health Affairs* 30, no. 1 (2011): 91–99, https://www.healthaffairs.org/doi/10.1377/hlthaff.2009.1087, https://doi.org/10.1377/hlthaff.2009.1087.

27. Susan Morse, "Medicare Proposed Changes Would Cut Home Health Reimbursement," *Healthcare Finance News*, July 26, 2017, http://www.healthcarefinancenews.com/news/home-health-agencies-concerned-about-cuts-proposed-medicare-payments.

28. Victoria Craig Bunce and J. P. Wieske, "Health Insurance Mandates in the States 2009: A State-by-State Breakdown of Health Insurance Mandates and Their Costs," Council for Affordable Health Insurance, 2009, https://www2.cbia.com/ieb/ag/CostOfCare/RisingCosts/CAHI_HealthInsuranceMandates2009.pdf.

29. "In the United States, Which Has a Greater Percentage of Fraud Committed: Medicare/Medicaid or Private Insurance?" Quora, https://www.quora.com/In-the-United-States-which-has-a-greater-percentage-of-fraud-committed-Medicare-Medicaid-or-private-insurance, accessed February 10, 2018.

30. Jim Avila, Serena Marshall, and Gitika Kaul, "Medicare Funds Totaling $60 Billion Improperly Paid, Report Finds," ABC News, July 23, 2015, http://abcnews.go.com/Politics/medicare-funds-totaling-60-billion-improperly-paid-report/story?id=32604330.

31. "Health Care Fraud: Types of Providers Involved in Medicare, Medicaid, and the Children's Health Insurance Program Cases; What GAO Found," Report to Congressional Requesters, United States Government Accounting Office, September 2012, https://www.gao.gov/assets/650/647849.pdf.

32. Atul Gawande, "The Cost Conundrum: What a Texas Town Can Teach Us about Health Care," *The New Yorker*, June 1, 2009, https://www.newyorker.com/magazine/2009/06/01/the-cost-conundrum.

33. Luisa Franzini, Osama I. Mikhail, and Jonathan S. Skinner, "McAllen and El Paso Revisited: Medicare Variations Not Always Reflected in the Under-Sixty-Five Population," *Health Affairs* 29, no. 12 (2010): 2302–9, https://www.healthaffairs.org/doi/10.1377/hlthaff.2010.0492, doi:10.1377/hlthaff.2010.0492.

34. Tracie L. Thompson, "Automated Claim Coding Pays Off in Time and Money," *Aunt-Minnie.com*, May 11, 2004, https://www.auntminnie.com/index.aspx?sec=ser&sub=def&pag=dis&ItemID=61697.

35. Jacqueline Fox, "Medicare Should, but Cannot, Consider Cost: Legal Impediments to a Sound Policy," *Buffalo Law Review* 53 (2005), http://scholarcommons.sc.edu/law_facpub, accessed February 10, 2018.

36. Ben Hirschler, "How the U.S. Pays 3 Times More for Drugs," Reuters, *Scientific American*, https://www.scientificamerican.com/article/how-the-u-s-pays-3-times-more-for-drugs/; Panos Kanavos, Alessandra Ferrario, Sotiris Vandoros, and Gerard F. Anderson, "Higher US Branded Drug Prices and Spending Compared to Other Countries May Stem Partly from Quick Uptake of New Drugs," *Health Affairs* 32, no. 4 (2013): 753–61, https://www.healthaffairs.org/doi/10.1377/hlthaff.2012.0920, doi:10.1377/hlthaff.2012.0920.

37. "Social Value Judgements: Principles for the Development of NICE Guidelines," 2nd ed., National Institute for Health and Clinical Excellence, accessed March 25, 2019, https://www.nice.org.uk/Media/Default/About/what-we-do/Research-and-development/Social-Value-Judgements-principles-for-the-development-of-NICE-guidance.pdf.

38. Peter R. Orszag, "Issues Regarding Drug Price Negotiation in Medicare," letter to the Honorable Ron Wyden, Congressional Budget Office, April 10, 2007, https://www.cbo.gov/sites/default/files/110th-congress-2007-2008/reports/drugpricenegotiation.pdf.

39. Luke Slawomirski, Ane Auraaen, and Niek Klazinga, "The Economics of Patient Safety: Strengthening a Value-Based Approach to Reducing Patient Harm at National Level," Organisation for Economic Co-operation and Development, March 2017, https://www.oecd.org/els/health-systems/The-economics-of-patient-safety-March-2017.pdf.

40. Roger Watson, "Could Super Nurses Make Up for the Shortfall in Doctors?" *The Independent*, April 13, 2017, http://www.independent.co.uk/life-style/health-and-families/could-super-nurses-make-up-for-the-shortfall-in-doctors-a7682091.html.

41. Michael K. Ong, Patrick S. Romano, Sarah Edgington, Harriet U. Aronow, Andrew D. Auerbach, Jeanne T. Black, Teresa De Marco, et al., "Effectiveness of Remote Patient Monitoring after Discharge of Hospitalized Patients with Heart Failure: The Better Effectiveness after Transition–Heart Failure (BEAT-HF) Randomized Clinical Trial," *JAMA Internal Medicine* 176, no. 3 (2016): 310, https://jamanetwork.com/journals/jamainternalmedicine/fullarticle/2488923, doi:10.1001/jamainternmed.2015.7712.

42. Brett D. Stauffer, Cliff Fullerton, Neil Fleming, Gerald Ogala, Jeph Herrin, Pamela Martin Stafford, and David J. Ballard, "Effectiveness and Cost of a Transitional Care Program for Heart Failure: A Prospective Study with Concurrent Controls," *Archives of Internal Medicine* 171, no. 14 (2011): 1238, https://jamanetwork.com/journals/jamainternalmedicine/fullarticle/1105852, doi:10.1001/archinternmed.2011.274.

43. S. Craig Thomas, Robert A. Greevy, and Arthur Garson Jr., "Effect of Grand-Aides Nurse Extenders on Readmissions and Emergency Department Visits in Medicare Patients with Heart Failure," *American Journal of Cardiology* 121, no. 11 (2018): 1336–42, https://www.ajconline.org/article/S0002-9149(18)30248-0/fulltext, doi:10.1016/j.amjcard.2018.02.012.

44. Robin Weinick and Renée Betancourt, "No Appointment Needed: The Resurgence of Urgent Care Centers in the United States," California Health Care Foundation (website), September 17, 2017, https://www.chcf.org/publication/no-appointment-needed-the-resurgence-of-urgent-care-centers-in-the-united-states/.

45. Robin M. Weinick, Rachel M. Burns, and Ateev Mehrotra, "Many Emergency Department Visits Could Be Managed at Urgent Care Centers and Retail Clinics," *Health Affairs* 29, no. 9 (2010): 1630–36, https://www.healthaffairs.org/doi/10.1377/hlthaff.2009.0748, doi: 10.1377/hlthaff.2009.0748.

46. "Study: 71% of ED Visits Unnecessary, Avoidable," Becker's Hospital Review, April 25, 2013, https://www.beckershospitalreview.com/patient-flow/study-71-of-ed-visits-unnecessary-avoidable.html; Arthur Garson, Donna M. Green, Lia Rodriguez, Richard Beech, and Christopher Nye, "A New Corps of Trained Grand-Aides Has the Potential to Extend Reach of Primary Care Workforce and Save Money," *Health Affairs* 31, no. 5 (2012): 1016–21, https://www.healthaffairs.org/doi/full/10.1377/hlthaff.2011.0859, doi:10.1377/hlthaff.2011.0859.

47. Sarah Kliff and German Lopez, "Obamacare's Changes to Doctor Payments, Explained," *Vox*, updated May 13, 2015, https://www.vox.com/cards/how-doctors-are-paid/bend-the-health-care-cost-curve.

48. Ezekiel J. Emanuel, "Are Hospitals Becoming Obsolete?" *New York Times*, February 25, 2018, https://www.nytimes.com/2018/02/25/opinion/hospitals-becoming-obsolete.html.

## 17. MYTH: WHEN IT COMES RIGHT DOWN TO IT, AMERICANS ARE LIKE EVERYONE ELSE

1. "Six in Ten Prefer to Be British than of Any Country on Earth," Ipsos MORI (website), September 9, 2016, https://www.ipsos.com/ipsos-mori/en-uk/six-ten-prefer-be-british-any-country-earth.

2. Mark Sappenfield, "Opening Ceremony London 2012: Did Director Take Shot at US on Health Care?" *Christian Science Monitor*, July 28, 2012, https://www.csmonitor.com/World/Olympics/2012/0728/Opening-Ceremony-London-2012-Did-director-take-shot-at-US-on-health-care.

3. T. R. Reid, "Five Myths about Health Care in the Rest of the World," *Washington Post*, August 23, 2009, http://www.washingtonpost.com/wp-dyn/content/article/2009/08/21/AR2009082101778.html.

4. Arthur Garson and Carolyn L. Engelhard, "Are We There Yet?" *Governing*, December 8, 2009, http://www.governing.com/topics/health-human-services/Are-We-There-Yet.html.

5. "Key Facts about the Uninsured Population," Henry J. Kaiser Family Foundation (website), December 7, 2018, https://www.kff.org/uninsured/fact-sheet/key-facts-about-the-uninsured-population/.

6. Michael Koren, "How Does the Government Protect the Rights of Its Citizens?" *eNotes*, https://www.enotes.com/homework-help/how-government-protect-rights-its-citizens-504866, accessed October 9, 2018.

7. K. M. Ho, K. Y. Lee, T. Williams, J. Finn, M. Knuiman, and S. A. R. Webb, "Comparison of Acute Physiology and Chronic Health Evaluation (APACHE) II Score with Organ Failure Scores to Predict Hospital Mortality," *Anaesthesia* 62, no. 5 (2007): 466–73, retrieved from https://onlinelibrary.wiley.com/doi/full/10.1111/j.1365-2044.2007.04999.x, doi:10.1111/j.1365-2044.2007.04999.x.

8. Suzanne Rivecca, *Death Is Not an Option: Stories* (New York and London: W. W. Norton, 2010).

9. Jerry Jasinowski, "It's the Economy, Stupid," *Huffington Post*, November 5, 2016, https://www.huffingtonpost.com/jerry-jasinowski/presidential-debates_b_8478456.html.

10. Michael Graham, "Commentary: 'It's the Economy, Stupid' Could Be Trumped," CBS News, January 25, 2015, https://www.cbsnews.com/news/commentary-its-the-economy-stupid-could-be-trumped/.

11. Madison Park, "Here's How Many Would Be Uninsured in Each Health Care Scenario," CNN, July 18, 2017, https://edition.cnn.com/2017/07/18/politics/health-care-options-unin sured/index.html.

12. Arthur Garson and David Blumenthal, "State-Federal Partnerships for Access to Care," *Journal of the American Medical Association* 297, no. 10 (2007): 1112–15, doi:10.1001/jama.297.10.1112.

13. "Health: Summary: Sector Profile, 2018," *OpenSecrets.org*, data downloaded January 24, 2019, https://www.opensecrets.org/lobby/indus.php?id=H.

14. "American Medical Assn: Summary: 2018," *OpenSecrets.org*, data downloaded January 24, 2019, https://www.opensecrets.org/lobby/clientsum.php?id=D000000068&year=2018.

15. Arthur Garson and David Blumenthal, "State-Federal Partnerships for Access to Care," *Journal of the American Medical Association* 297, no. 10 (2007): 1112–15, doi:10.1001/jama.297.10.1112.

16. Thom File, "Voting in America: A Look at the 2016 Presidential Election," *Census Blogs*, United States Census Bureau, May 10, 2017, https://www.census.gov/newsroom/blogs/random-samplings/2017/05/voting_in_america.html.

# 18. MYTH: PREVIOUS ATTEMPTS AT HEALTH-CARE REFORM HAVE TAUGHT US VERY LITTLE

1. Matthew Caleb Flamm, s.v. "George Santayana (1863–1952)," *Internet Encyclopedia of Philosophy*, https://www.iep.utm.edu/santayan/, accessed November 14, 2018.

2. Jonathan Oberlander, "Unfinished Journey—A Century of Health Care Reform in the United States," *New England Journal of Medicine* 367, no. 7 (2012): 585–90, https://www.nejm.org/doi/full/10.1056/nejmp1202111, doi:10.1056/NEJMp1202111.

3. Clinton's plan culminated in the Health Security Act, H.R. 3600, 103rd Cong. (1993–1994), text available at https://www.congress.gov/bill/103rd-congress/house-bill/3600/text.

4. Adam Clymer, Robert Pear, and Robin Toner, "The Health Care Debate: What Went Wrong? How the Health Care Campaign Collapsed: A Special Report; For Health Care, Times Was a Killer," *New York Times*, August 29, 1994, http://www.nytimes.com/1994/08/29/us/health-care-debate-what-went-wrong-health-care-campaign-collapsed-special-report.html?pagewanted=all.

5. Alain C. Enthoven, "The History and Principles of Managed Competition," *Health Affairs* 12, no. supplement 1 (1993): 24–48, https://www.healthaffairs.org/doi/10.1377/hlthaff.12.Suppl_1.24, doi:10.1377/hlthaff.12.suppl_1.24.

6. Robert Pear, "Clinton's Health Plan: The Overview; Congress Is Given Clinton Proposal for Health Care," *New York Times*, October 28, 1993, http://www.nytimes.com/1993/10/28/us/

clinton-s-health-plan-overview-congress-given-clinton-proposal-for-health-care.html?page
wanted=all.

7. Robert Moffit, "A Guide to the Clinton Health Plan," Heritage Foundation (website), November 19, 1993, https://www.heritage.org/health-care-reform/report/guide-the-clinton-health-plan.

8. "12 Simply Stated Features of the Affordable Care Act/Obamacare," *Health Power for Minorities*, accessed March 6, 2018, http://healthpowerforminorities.com/12-simply-stated-features-of-the-affordable-care-act/.

9. Richard S. Foster, "Estimated Financial Effects of the 'Patient Protection and Affordable Care Act,' as Amended," Centers for Medicare and Medicaid Services, April 22, 2010, https://www.cms.gov/Research-Statistics-Data-and-Systems/Research/ActuarialStudies/downloads/PPACA_2010-04-22.pdf.

10. "Prior HHS Poverty Guidelines and Federal Register References," Office of the Assistant Secretary for Planning and Evaluation (website), https://aspe.hhs.gov/prior-hhs-poverty-guidelines-and-federal-register-references, accessed November 14, 2018.

11. "10 Essential Health Benefits Insurance Plans Must Cover Under the Affordable Care Act," *Families USA* (blog), February 9, 2018, https://familiesusa.org/blog/10-essential-health-benefits-insurance-plans-must-cover, accessed October 9, 2018.

12. "Closing the Medicare Part D Donut Hole," National Committee to Protect Social Security and Medicare (website), June 28, 2016, https://www.ncpssm.org/documents/general-archives-2016/closing-the-medicare-part-d-donut-hole/.

13. Alicia Adamczyk, "5 Things to Know about AHCA, the New Republican Health Care Bill that Just Passed," *Money*, May 4, 2017, http://time.com/money/4766063/ahca-new-republican-health-care-bill/.

14. Robert Pear, "What's in the AHCA: The Major Provisions of the Republican Health Bill," *New York Times*, May 4, 2017, https://www.nytimes.com/2017/05/04/us/politics/major-provisions-republican-health-care-bill.html.

15. Robin A. Cohen, Diane M. Makuc, Amy B. Bernstein, Linda T. Bilheimer, and Eve Powell-Griner, "Health Insurance Coverage Trends, 1959–2007: Estimates from the National Health Interview Survey," *National Health Statistics Reports*, July 1, 2009, no. 17, https://www.cdc.gov/nchs/data/nhsr/nhsr017.pdf.

16. Gretchen Jacobson, Tricia Neuman, and MaryBeth Musumeci, "What Could a Medicaid Per Capita Cap Mean for Low-Income People on Medicare?" Henry J. Kaiser Family Foundation (website), March 24, 2017, https://www.kff.org/medicare/issue-brief/what-could-a-medicaid-per-capita-cap-mean-for-low-income-people-on-medicare/.

17. Simon Maloy, "GOP's Health Care Tax Swindle: Tax Cuts for the Rich Financed by Taking Coverage from Everyone Else," *Salon*, March 9, 2017, https://www.salon.com/2017/03/09/gops-health-care-tax-swindle-tax-cuts-for-the-rich-financed-by-taking-coverage-from-everyone-else/.

18. Arthur "Tim" Garson, Stephen H. Linder, and Ryan Holeywell, "The Nation's Pulse: The Texas Medical Center's Customer & Physician Survey," slides of survey findings, Texas Medical Center, 2017, https://www.tmc.edu/health-policy/wp-content/uploads/sites/5/2017/09/2017NationsPulsePresentation.pdf.

19. Tara O'Neill Hayes, "Alternative Policy Options to the Individual Mandate," American Action Forum (website), June 20, 2017, https://www.americanactionforum.org/insight/alternative-policy-options-individual-mandate/.

20. Arthur Garson and David Blumenthal, "State-Federal Partnerships for Access to Care," *Journal of the American Medical Association* 297, no. 10 (2007): 1112–15, doi:10.1001/jama.297.10.1112.

# 19. MYTH: AMERICANS ARE SO DIVIDED THAT WE CAN'T EVEN AGREE ON GOALS FOR OUR HEALTH CARE

1. Arthur Garson Jr., "President's Page: The U.S. Healthcare System 2010; Problems, Principles, and Potential Solutions," *Journal of the American College of Cardiology* 35, no. 4 (2000): 1048–52, http://www.onlinejacc.org/content/35/4/1048, doi:10.1016/S0735-1097(00) 00569-6.

2. Melanie Schoenberg, Natalie Chau, David Salsberry, and Allen Miller, "Delivery System Reform in Section 1115 Waivers: A Texas Experience," Region 10 Health Partnership (RHP) for the Texas 1115 Medicaid Waiver (website), http://www.rhp10txwaiver.com/images/ Delivery_System_Reform_in_Section_1115_Waivers_-_A_Texas_Experience.pdf, accessed February 11, 2018.

3. "UVA Health System: The Wise Remote Area Medical (RAM) Program," American Hospital Association (website), April 18, 2012, https://aha.org/case-studies/2012-04-18-uva-health-system-wise-remote-area-medical-ram-program.

4. [Clinic schedule], Remote Area Medical (website), accessed March 8, 2018, https:// www.ramusa.org/clinic-schedule/.

5. John Graves, Pranita Mishra, Robert Dittus, Ravi Parikh, Jennifer Perloff, and Peter Buerhaus, "Role of Geography and Nurse Practitioner Scope-of-Practice in Efforts to Expand Primary Care System Capacity: Health Reform and the Primary Care Workforce," *Medical Care* 54, no. 1 (2016): 81–89, doi:10.1097/MLR.0000000000000454.

6. Robert Wood Johnson Foundation and the Institute of Medicine, *The Future of Nursing: Leading Change, Advancing Health* (Washington, DC: National Academies Press, 2010).

7. Keith Carlson, "NP Practice Authority Grows: March 2017 Update," Nurse.org, March 2, 2017, https://nurse.org/articles/nurse-practitioner-scope-of-practice-expands-mar17/.

8. Mariana Alfaro, "Texas Nurse Practitioners Again Push for Independence," *Texas Tribune*, February 9, 2017, https://www.texastribune.org/2017/02/09/nurse-practitioners-push-independence-once-again/.

9. John Graves, Pranita Mishra, Robert Dittus, Ravi Parikh, Jennifer Perloff, and Peter Buerhaus, "Role of Geography and Nurse Practitioner Scope-of-Practice in Efforts to Expand Primary Care System Capacity: Health Reform and the Primary Care Workforce," *Medical Care* 54, no. 1 (2016): 81–89, doi:10.1097/MLR.0000000000000454.

10. Jennifer Perloff, Catherine M. DesRoches, and Peter Buerhaus, "Comparing the Cost of Care Provided to Medicare Beneficiaries Assigned to Primary Care Nurse Practitioners and Physicians," *Health Services Research* 51, no. 4 (2016): 1407–23, doi:10.1111/1475-6773 .12425.

11. Joseph P. Williams, "Wanted: Rural Doctors; In Alabama and Elsewhere in the U.S., a Physician Shortage Feeds Community Ills," Healthiest Communities, US News and World Report, August 22, 2018, https://www.usnews.com/news/healthiest-communities/articles/2018-08-22/rural-doctor-shortage-a-drag-on-community-health.

12. Anne Cantrell, "MSU Study Finds Nurse Practitioners More Likely than Medical Doctors to Work in Rural Areas," Montana State University (website), January 14, 2016, http:// www.montana.edu/news/15928/msu-study-finds-nurse-practitioners-more-likely-than-medical-doctors-to-work-in-rural-areas.

13. Arthur Garson, "Grand-Aides and Health Policy: Reducing Readmissions Cost-Effectively," *Health Affairs Blog*, October 29, 2014, https://www.healthaffairs.org/do/10.1377/hblog20141029.041916/full/.

14. Christal Ramos, Terri Coughlin, Adam Weiss, and Sharon K. Long, "Federally Qualified Health Center Users Continue to Have Limited Options for Health Care under Health Reform and Give Federally Qualified Health Centers Mixed Reviews," *Health Reform Monitoring Survey*, Urban Institute Health Policy Center, http://hrms.urban.org/briefs/federally-qualified-health-centers-options-reviews.html.

15. Arthur "Tim" Garson, Stephen H. Linder, and Ryan Holeywell, "The Nation's Pulse: The Texas Medical Center's Customer & Physician Survey," slides of survey findings, Texas Medical Center, 2017, https://www.tmc.edu/health-policy/wp-content/uploads/sites/5/2017/09/2017NationsPulsePresentation.pdf.

16. "More than Half of Consumers Now Buy on Their Beliefs," Edelman (website), June 8, 2017, https://www.edelman.com/news-awards/consumers-now-buy-on-beliefs-2017-earned-brand.

17. We originally published this section as an op-ed, as Arthur "Tim" Garson Jr., "Dear Alex Azar: The Next HHS Secretary Must Redefine 'Affordable' Health Care," November 14, 2017, *STAT*, https://www.statnews.com/2017/11/14/alex-azar-affordable-health-care/.

18. "ACA'S Affordability Contribution Percentage Increase for 2017," Horton Group, May 3, 2016, https://www.thehortongroup.com/resources/acas-affordability-contribution-percentage-increase-for-2017.

19. Lola Butcher, "Shared Decision-Making: Giving the Patient a Say. No, Really," *Hospitals and Health Networks Magazine*, May 1, 2013, https://www.hhnmag.com/articles/6284-shared-decision-making-giving-the-patient-a-say-no-really.

20. Donald M. Berwick and Andrew D. Hackbarth, "Eliminating Waste in US Health Care," *Journal of the American Medical Association* 307, no. 14 (2012): 1513, doi:10.1001/jama.2012.362.

21. T. Gosden, L. Pedersen, and D. Torgerson, "How Should We Pay Doctors? A Systematic Review of Salary Payments and Their Effect on Doctor Behaviour," *QJM* 92, no. 1 (1999): 47–55, https://academic.oup.com/qjmed/article/92/1/47/1550410, doi:10.1093/qjmed/92.1.47; J. Broomberg and M. R. Price, "The Impact of the Fee-for-Service Reimbursement System on the Utilisation of Health Services. Part II. Comparison of Utilisation Patterns in Medical Aid Schemes and a Local Health Maintenance Organisation," *South African Medical Journal* 78, no. 3 (1990): 133–36; Willard G. Manning, Arleen Leibowitz, George A. Goldberg, William H. Rogers, and Joseph P. Newhouse, "A Controlled Trial of the Effect of a Prepaid Group Practice on Use of Services," *New England Journal of Medicine* 310, no. 23 (1984): 1505–10, doi:10.1056/NEJM198406073102305.

22. Joanne Finnegan, "Survey Finds Many Doctors Prefer Being Paid a Salary Instead of Per Volume," *FierceHealthcare*, September 19, 2017, https://www.fiercehealthcare.com/practices/survey-finds-many-doctors-prefer-being-paid-a-salary.

23. S.v. "Capitation vs. Fee for Service," *Diffen*, https://www.diffen.com/difference/Capitation_vs_Fee_For_Service, accessed February 11, 2018.

24. Heather Landi, "Physician Survey: EHRs Increase Practice Costs, Reduce Productivity," *Healthcare Informatics Magazine*, October 3, 2016, https://www.healthcare-informatics.com/news-item/ehr/physician-survey-ehrs-increase-practice-costs-little-improvement-clinical-outcomes.

25. Andrew Gottschalk and Susan A. Flocke, "Time Spent with Patient Care versus Administrative Work," *Medscape*, 2016.

26. Donald M. Berwick and Andrew D. Hackbarth, "Eliminating Waste in US Health Care," *Journal of the American Medical Association* 307, no. 14 (2012): 1513, doi:10.1001/jama.2012.362.

27. "Conflating Costs of the ACA," *FactCheck.org*, February 6, 2015, https://www.factcheck.org/2015/02/conflating-costs-of-the-aca/.

28. Arthur Garson, "Grand-Aides and Health Policy: Reducing Readmissions Cost-Effectively," *Health Affairs Blog*, October 29, 2014, https://www.healthaffairs.org/do/10.1377/hblog20141029.041916/full/; S. Craig Thomas, Robert A. Greevy, and Arthur Garson, "Effect of Grand-Aides Nurse Extenders on Readmissions and Emergency Department Visits in Medicare Patients with Heart Failure," *American Journal of Cardiology* 121, no. 11 (2018): 1336–42, https://www.ajconline.org/article/S0002-9149(18)30248-0/fulltext, doi:10.1016/j.amjcard.2018.02.012.

29. "Life Expectancy for Countries," *World Factbook*, US Central Intelligence Agency, 2015, available at https://www.infoplease.com/world/health-and-social-statistics/life-expectancy-countries-0.

# 20. MYTH: THERE IS NO HEALTH-CARE SYSTEM THAT WILL WORK FOR THE UNITED STATES

1. Letty Carpenter, "Special Report: Medicaid Eligibility for Persons in Nursing Homes," *Health Care Financing Review* 10, no. 2 (1988): 67–77, https://www.cms.gov/Research-Statistics-Data-and-Systems/Research/HealthCareFinancingReview/Downloads/CMS11910 21dl.pdf.

2. Niccolò Machiavelli, from the English translation of chapter 6 of *Il Principe* [*The Prince*] (1532).

3. Danielle Kurtzleben, "Bernie Sanders' 'Medicare for All' Bill: Here's What It Would Do," NPR, September 14, 2017, https://www.npr.org/2017/09/14/550768280/heres-whats-in-bernie-sanders-medicare-for-all-bill.

4. CAP Health Policy Team, "Medicare Extra for All," Center for American Progress (website), February 22, 2018, https://www.americanprogress.org/issues/healthcare/reports/2018/02/22/447095/medicare-extra-for-all/.

5. Patrick Collinson, "Private Health Insurance Sales Surge amid NHS Crisis," *The Guardian*, January 15, 2017, https://www.theguardian.com/business/2017/jan/16/private-medical-insurance-sales-surge-health-nhs.

6. Mollyann Brodie, Elizabeth C. Hamel, and Mira Norton, "Medicare as Reflected in Public Opinion," *American Society on Aging* (blog), https://www.asaging.org/blog/medicare-reflected-public-opinion, accessed November 17, 2018.

7. Ryan Whitacker, "How Much Universal Healthcare Would Cost in the US," *Decision Data*, November 11, 2015, https://decisiondata.org/news/how-much-single-payer-uhc-would-cost-usa/.

8. Arthur Garson and David Blumenthal, "State-Federal Partnerships for Access to Care," *Journal of the American Medical Association* 297, no. 10 (2007): 1112-15, doi:10.1001/jama.297.10.1112.

9. Mary Agnes Carey, "Lawmakers Unveil Bill that Would Help Fund States' Efforts to Cover Uninsured," Commonwealth Fund (website), January 17, 2007, https://www.

commonwealthfund.org/publications/newsletter-article/lawmakers-unveil-bill-would-help-fund-states-efforts-cover.

## FINAL WORDS

1. Carl Sagan, *The Demon-Haunted World: Science as a Candle in the Dark* (New York: Random House, 1995), 12.

# Index

# About the Authors

**Arthur Garson Jr.**, MD, MPH (also known as "Tim"), is director of the Health Policy Institute at the Texas Medical Center in Houston, home to sixty-one members, including twenty-six hospitals and four medical schools. He has more than forty years of experience as a practicing pediatric cardiologist. After serving as chief of pediatric cardiology at the renowned Texas Children's Hospital, he was associate vice-chancellor for health policy at Duke University and then was recruited back to Houston to serve at Texas Children's as vice president of quality and as dean of academic operations at Baylor College of Medicine. He was then dean at the University of Virginia's School of Medicine before becoming provost for all of UVA. He returned to Houston for his current position. He has been president of the American College of Cardiology, as well as chair of the National Advisory Council for Healthcare Research and Quality, and is an elected member of the National Academy of Sciences' National Academy of Medicine (Institute of Medicine).

Why the shift from pediatric cardiology to health policy? He witnessed firsthand what happens when we have bad health policy. Early in his career, he began treating a five-year-old girl named Virginia (Ginny for short). The night he first started caring for her, she arrested three times after open-heart surgery but eventually made it through after a rocky start. Garson became Ginny's doctor and bonded with the entire family—even attending Ginny's grammar school and high school graduations.

Ginny developed a hearth-rhythm problem that could easily be controlled with medication but would be fatal without it. During the summer of Ginny's nineteenth year, her mother called Garson and delivered the horrible news: Ginny had been found dead in her bedroom. It turned out that Ginny hadn't refilled any of her four heart-medication prescriptions. She was no longer eligible for Medicaid, the state-run insurance program for the poor. Ginny's death had a profound effect on Garson. He shifted his career to focus on how we could develop better health policy in order to fix the problem of the uninsured and prevent other people from dying a needless death the way Ginny did.

**Ryan Holeywell** spent more than a decade as a journalist working in Washington, D.C., and Texas, but his very first full-time job was working as a newspaper reporter in McAllen, Texas, a city of 140,000 on the United States–Mexico border and one of poorest communities in the country. During his time there, Holeywell saw firsthand the link between poverty, health, and lack of insurance. More than 30 percent of residents living in and around McAllen have diabetes, compared to 12 percent of US residents. Similarly, the region's obesity rate is among the worst in the country, which has drawn national attention. Even with the strides that have been made in the wake of the Affordable Care Act, a third of residents under the age of sixty-five in that region are still uninsured. It struck Holeywell as fundamentally unfair that in a nation that invests tens of billions of dollars in medical research every year, McAllen residents suffer because they had the bad fortunate to be born poor in the wrong part of the country.

The community also had the dubious distinction of being featured in a famous *New Yorker* article that identified the region as having the second-highest Medicare expenses in the country, despite the extremely low cost of living, because of "across-the-board overuse of medicine" and the "entrepreneurial spirit" of the area's doctors. One could argue that the extreme health disparities in McAllen, along with those exorbitant costs, make it a microcosm for everything wrong with American health care.

After working in McAllen, Holeywell eventually became a reporter in Washington, D.C., where he frequently interviewed members of Congress, cabinet officials, governors, and mayors from across the country as a reporter for *Governing* magazine, which focuses on trends in state and local governments. Far from leaving him cynical (as D.C. reporting stints can do), the experience left him hopeful that even in the face of inaction in Washington, some lawmakers—especially those in state and local government—are eager to take on many of the country's biggest challenges, including health care.

Holeywell has also worked as a business reporter for the *Houston Chronicle*, and he has appeared on CNN, NPR, and CNBC to discuss his work. Today he leads communications at the Texas Medical Center in Houston.